The SAGES Manual Ethics of Surgical Innovation

Steven C. Stain • Aurora D. Pryor
Phillip P. Shadduck

Editors

The SAGES Manual Ethics of Surgical Innovation

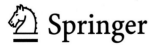 Springer

Editors
Steven C. Stain
Department of Surgery
Albany Medical College
Albany, NY, USA

Aurora D. Pryor
Division of General Surgery
Stony Brook School of Medicine
Stony Brook, NY, USA

Phillip P. Shadduck
Department of Surgery
Triangle Orthopaedic Associates
Durham, NC, USA

ISBN 978-3-319-27661-8   ISBN 978-3-319-27663-2   (eBook)
DOI 10.1007/978-3-319-27663-2

Library of Congress Control Number: 2016936896

Printed on acid-free paper

This Springer imprint is published by Springer Nature
The registered company is Springer International Publishing AG Switzerland

Foreword

Innovation is the way forward in surgery. Without the possibility to do things differently, surgeons would continue to care for patients today the way that they did a century ago. However, it is clear that not all new ideas in surgery are good ideas. It is through creative attempts by surgeons to solve patient problems that innovations in surgery arise.

The ethics of innovation is ultimately a test of the ethical behavior of surgeons. It is up to surgeons to identify creative solutions to their patients' problems, and it is up to surgeons whether to offer to use innovative techniques in their care of patients. Surgeons are responsible for avoiding or managing potential conflicts of interest that may negatively affect their patients. Surgeons are also the central parties in informing their patients about new techniques and technologies and ensuring adequate consent from their patients.

Surgeons play a central role in all aspects of innovation. This fact makes the new SAGES Manual on the *Ethics of Surgical Innovation* so critically important. Surgeons must be attentive to the ethical issues in surgical innovation and they must play a central role in ensuring that innovations are implemented in an ethical manner. This volume will go a long way toward guaranteeing that the ethical issues in surgical innovation are given the level of attention in future years that they warrant. It is gratifying that surgeons have taken the ethical aspects of surgical innovation so seriously that a volume such as this is possible.

MacLean Center for Clinical Medical Ethics   Peter Angelos
The University of Chicago
Chicago, IL, USA

Preface

Surgeons have been leaders in the development of new therapies and technologies for generations. Surgeon innovators are critical partners in surgical device development—to discover unmet needs, to shepherd the new product development process, to design and conduct clinical trials, to establish evidence-based and financially responsible clinical guidelines, and to define training and credentialing processes. Yet, participating in innovation creates a number of ethical issues that must be recognized and managed wisely by the physicians—relationships with industry partners, necessary for device development, regulatory approval, manufacturing, and marketing; relationships with investors and corporations who provide the millions of dollars required to bring a product to market; and relationships with patients, especially those who "go first," who deserve to know the role that the surgeon had in the development of the product and what financial gain he/she may receive from the product. Additionally, many new technologies or therapies are more expensive than their predecessors. Insurance companies, federal healthcare programs, and the public will ultimately bear the cost of newer therapies, and these payors need to have a mechanism for the evaluating and adopting innovative treatments.

The purpose of this manual is to review the many ethical issues involved in the development, evaluation, and introduction of new treatments for gastrointestinal diseases. We have asked recognized surgical innovators to describe how several landmark procedures were developed in order to illustrate the challenges and ethical dilemmas that they struggled with. Selected chapters will explain how to work with industry partners and investors, and the challenges of dealing with increasing and uncertain regulatory issues. Once a new technology has been brought to the market, guidelines and standards need to be developed regarding the training, credentialing and adoption of the technology. There are often insufficient standards for balancing the desire to provide patients the latest therapy with the obligation to provide an appropriate and transparent informed consent process. These issues will also be addressed.

This manual was borne of two symposia at the Society of Gastrointestinal and Endoscopic Surgeons (SAGES) Annual Meeting, sessions that the editors were honored to host--Innovations in the Era of Conflict of Interest and Transparency, and The Ethics of Innovation. We appreciate the encouragement of then SAGES President, Dr Gerald Fried, to proceed with this project. We are also indebted to the SAGES Board and staff for their tremendous support. We hope that these chapters will serve a resource for surgeons and other physician innovators, researchers and health policy personnel, the medical device industry, and university biodesign departments to better understand the ethical issues related to the development, introduction and adoption of innovative therapies.

Albany, NY, USA   Steven C. Stain
Stony Brook, NY, USA   Aurora D. Pryor
Durham, NC, USA   Phillip P. Shadduck
October 2015

Contents

Contributors

Rizwan Ahmed
Department of Surgery, Duke University School of Medicine, Durham, NC, USA

Department of Surgery, Johns Hopkins University School of Medicine, Baltimore, MD, USA

Maria S. Altieri
Division of Bariatric, Foregut and Advanced Gastrointestinal Surgery, Department of Surgery, Stony Brook University Medical Center, Stony Brook, NY, USA

Chady Atallah
Department of Surgery, Johns Hopkins University School of Medicine, Baltimore, MD, USA

Dan Azagury
Department of Surgery, Stanford University Medical Center, Biodesign Program, Stanford University, Stanford, CA, USA

Martha W. Betz
Center for Devices and Radiological Health, Food and Drug Administration, Silver Spring, MD, USA

Juliane Bingener
Department of Surgery, Mayo Clinic, Rochester, MN, USA

Myriam J. Curet
Intuitive Surgical, Sunnyvale, CA, USA

Stanford University, Stanford, CA, USA

Richard Dal Col
Medical Affairs, Capital District Physicians' Health Plan, Albany, NY, USA

Meredith C. Duke
Department of Surgery, University of North Carolina, Chapel Hill, NC, USA

David W. Easter
Department of Surgery, UC San Diego School of Medicine, La Jolla, CA, USA

Robert D. Fanelli
Division of Minimally Invasive Surgery and Surgical Endoscopy, Department of Surgery, The Guthrie Clinic, Sayre, PA, USA

Timothy M. Farrell
Department of Surgery, University of North Carolina, Chapel Hill, NC, USA

Luke C. Gelinas
Petrie-Flom Center for Health Law Policy, Biotechnology, and Bioethics, Harvard Law School, Cambridge, MA, USA

Caitlin Halbert
Division of Bariatric, Foregut and Advanced Gastrointestinal Surgery. Department of Surgery, Stony Brook University Medical Center, Stony Brook, NY, USA

Christiana Healthcare System, Dover, Delaware

John G. Hunter
Department of Surgery, Oregon Health & Science University, Portland, OR, USA

Tazo Inui
Vascular Surgery, Department of Surgery, UC San Diego, San Diego, CA, USA

Mudit K. Jain
Synergy Life Science Partners, Portola Valley, CA, USA

Crystal M. Krause
The Center for Advanced Surgical Technology, Department of Surgery, University of Nebraska Medical Center, Omaha, NE, USA

Thomas Krummel
Department of Surgery, Stanford University School of Medicine, Stanford, CA, USA

Division of Pediatric Surgery, Lucile Packard Children's Hospital Stanford, Biodesign Program, Stanford University, Stanford, CA, USA

Herbert Lerner
Center for Devices and Radiological Health, Food and Drug Administration, Silver Spring, MD, USA

Anne O. Lidor
Department of Surgery, Johns Hopkins University School of Medicine, Baltimore, MD, USA

Department of Surgery, University of Wisconsin School of Medicine and Public Health, Baltimore, MD, USA

James Melton
Clinical Development Partners, Precision Clinical Management, Chapel Hill, NC, USA

Peter Nau
Department of Surgery, The University of Iowa Hospitals and Clinics, Iowa City, IA, USA

Dmitry Oleynikov
The Center for Advanced Surgical Technology, Department of Surgery, University of Nebraska Medical Center, Omaha, NE, USA

Raymond P. Onders
Department of Surgery, University Hospitals Case Medical Center, Case Western Reserve University School of Medicine, Cleveland, OH, USA

Jeffrey L. Ponsky
Cleveland Clinic Lerner College of Medicine, Case Western Reserve University, Cleveland, OH, USA

Aurora Pryor
Division of Bariatric, Foregut and Advanced Gastrointestinal Surgery, Department of Surgery, Stony Brook University Medical Center, Stony Brook, NY, USA

David W. Rattner
Division of Gastrointestinal and General Surgery, Department of Surgery, Massachusetts General Hospital, Boston, MA, USA

Arthur L. Rawlings
Department of Surgery, University of Missouri, Columbia, MO, USA

John H. Rodriguez
Department of General Surgery, Cleveland Clinic Foundation, Cleveland, OH, USA

C.J. Schwaitzberg
Northwestern University, Evanston, IL, USA

S.D. Schwaitzberg
Department of Surgery, University at Buffalo School of Medicine and Biomedical Sciences, Buffalo, NY, USA

Department of Surgery, Harvard Medical School, Cambridge Hospital, Cambridge, MA, USA

Phillip P. Shadduck
Department of Surgery, Triangle Orthopaedic Associates, Durham, NC, USA

Lelan F. Sillin
Department of Surgery, Lahey Hospital and Medical Center, Burlington, MA, USA

Richard S. Stack
Synergy Life Science Partners, San Francisco, CA, USA

Synecor, Chapel Hill, NC, USA

William N. Starling
Synergy Life Science Partners, San Francisco, CA, USA

Synecor, Chapel Hill, NC, USA

Donna Stewart
Medical Affairs, Capital District Physicians' Health Plan, Latham, NY, USA

Lee L. Swanström
Department of GI/MIS Surgery, The Oregon Clinic, Portland, OR, USA

IHU-Strasbourg, University of Strasbourg, Strasbourg, France

David R. Urbach
Department of Surgery, Institute of Health Policy, Management and Evaluation, University of Toronto, Toronto General Hospital, Toronto, ON, Canada

Jeffrey Ustin
Department of Biomedical Engineering, Case Western Reserve University, Cleveland, OH, USA

Department of Surgery, Akron General Medical Center, Akron, OH, USA

Gregory Van Stiegmann
Department of Surgery, GITES Division, University of Colorado Hospital, Aurora, CO, USA

Anji Wall
Department of General Surgery, Vanderbilt University, Nashville, TN, USA

James Wall
Division of Pediatric Surgery, Department of Surgery, Lucile Packard Children's Hospital Stanford, Biodesign Program, Stanford University, Palo Alto, CA, USA

Bruce D. White
Alden March Bioethics Institute, Albany Medical College, Albany, NY, USA

1. Historical Perspective of Surgical Innovation

John G. Hunter

From the beginning of time, surgeons demonstrated creativity and innovative thinking in approaching injury and illness, whether it be the gold plates discovered in the skulls of the Incas presumably to protect the brain after head injury or trephination, or the fine suture material of the Egyptians developed from natural fibers and discovered in mummies from 500 BC. In the English-speaking world, one generally traces innovation in surgery back to the founding of the first English-speaking College of Surgeons in Edinburgh, Scotland, in 1505. In the beginning, the surgeons were deeded not only the opportunity to advance the surgical cure of disease, the first charter deeded the rights to apothecary (pharmaceutical) development to the surgeons as well. While developments and innovations in pharmacology were passed over to the physicians and chemists rather early, initial surgical innovations revolved around the development of instruments that would allow the retrieval of bladder stones, ligation of peripheral aneurysms, phlebotomy, exploration of wounds, and amputation, a very limited spectrum of procedures before general anesthesia.

One hundred years years before the ether dome, the background for surgical experimentation and innovation was set in London by John and William Hunter and their many disciples. While William Hunter is best known as the obstetrician to the Royal Family, John Hunter was known as the anatomist and surgical scientist, who was often quoted as deriding textbooks in favor of experimentation and observation. To Edward Jenner in 1775, "I think your solution is just, but why think? Why not try the experiment?" The educational reach of Hunter came across the Atlantic Ocean with the two of their pupils who became the two surgeons to establish surgery in the first medical school in the United States, the University of Pennsylvania. John Morgan and Phillip Syng

© Springer International Publishing Switzerland 2016
S.C. Stain et al. (eds.), *The SAGES Manual Ethics
of Surgical Innovation*, DOI 10.1007/978-3-319-27663-2_1

Physick spent time in London learning the Hunterian principles in the late eighteenth century before returning to the USA to start a medical school in Philadelphia with Benjamin Rush, which would become the University of Pennsylvania, the oldest medical school in the United States.

The landmark innovation of the nineteenth century was the development of ether anesthesia, a story that started in Jefferson, Georgia, where Crawford Long first administered a general anesthesia in 1842 to the ether dome in Boston where William Morton grabbed history in 1846. Crawford Long's error was that he never published his development until 3 years after William Morton had cemented his place in history. Another lesson in innovation is publish your observations if you wish to get credit for the development.

Following the development of ether anesthesia, many operations were described and performed across Europe and the United States. Nonetheless, many of these were associated with life-threatening or lethal infections as Pasteur's work in understanding the biology of microbes was still in the test tube. While it was well known that infection killed more soldiers in the US Civil War than did swords or bullets that was soon to change. The US Civil Warth ended in 1865 and in that same year Joseph Lister, in Edinburgh, Scotland, started applying carbolic acid to open fractures before repair, dramatically reducing the rate of serious infection. Following these development in general anesthesia and sterile technique, the world of surgery took off. Many of the great developments and operations we perform commonly today were developed in a 20-year period from 1880 to 1900 by great innovators in Europe such as Billroth, Sauerbruch, Courvoisier, Kocher, Bassini, and Miles. In the USA, Halstead, Cushing, Mayo, Ochsner, Crile, and many others built upon the surgical developments of Europe, firmly putting the United States on the map as a center of surgical innovation. In the twentieth century, great surgical innovators pushed the boundaries with the developments of electrosurgery (Bovie and Cushing), open chest surgery (Churchill and Louis), vascular surgery (Bakey and Crawford), and open heart surgery (Lillihei, Gibbon, Starr, and Cooley). In the latter half of the twentieth century organ transplantation (Murray, Starzl, Barnard, Schumway) and parenteral nutrition (Dudrick and Rhodes) bolstered our ability to replace damaged organs and support patients through critical illnesses when the GI tract was not working.

The innovation that most changed general surgery in the last half century was the development of minimally invasive surgery, including flexible endoscopy, laparoscopy, thoracoscopy, and other image based modalities. The innovators in these fields are many, but Kurt Semm, George Berci, Eric Muhe, and a long line of others contributed to the developments in laparoscopic appendectomy, cholecystectomy, and many additional procedures.

Laparoscopy was an example of a disruptive innovation. Disruptive innovations are those technologies or techniques that are "game changers." The game is changed not by moving the football down the field but by changing the field entirely. The field was changed by the Hopkins rod-lens telescope, the fiberoptic endoscope, and the charge-coupled device (CCD) video camera that could be affixed to the viewing end of an endoscope. This technology was affordable, portable, and simple to use. When it was proven that common operations could be done with smaller incisions, less pain, and a shorter recovery—without adding cost or complications—the field of general surgery was forever different. Laparoscopy is one of many imaging modalities that allow minimally invasive procedures.

The other great advance of the late twentieth century was the development of fluoroscopic-assisted vascular intervention otherwise known as image-guided surgery or endovascular surgery. These developments can be largely attributed to Charlie Dotter, a radiologist in Oregon who was the first to perform dilation of an artery for the lower extremity ischemia in 1964. Dr. Dotter stated "An angiographic catheter can be more than a tool for passive means for diagnostic observation; usually the imagination, it can become an important surgical instrument."

Taxonomy of Innovation

Innovation can be described in various ways, but the simplest taxonomy divides innovation between that which is iterative or sustaining and that which is revolutionary or disruptive [1]. Earlier in this chapter, we introduced disruptive innovation as being nonlinear. Disruptive innovation starts when a new technology or new technique often from another field is introduced in a way that makes an established process cheaper, simpler, or more portable. While laparoscopy and image-guided surgery were two of the most disruptive influences in surgery over the last quarter century, other disruptive technologies and techniques are on the way. Hand-held portable ultra-sound units have already changed the game for central line placement where "blind" access to the central veins has been replaced by ultra-sound-guided puncture, reducing complications dramatically.

The other type of innovation, iterative or sustaining innovation, moves the football down the field. That is, problems in surgery are identified, and new instruments, devices, or techniques are adapted to improve performance. There are many examples of iterative innovation in our day-to-day lives as surgeons. For example, energy devices in surgery continue to evolve on an annual basis from standard electrosurgery to the harmonic scalpel to the Ligasure (Valley Labs, USA), and beyond. Tissue glue has replaced suture for closing small wounds. Vacuum-assisted wound closure devices have replaced frequent wound dressing changes as a means to manage the septic or edematous abdominal compartment, and so on. While disruptive innovations are certainly sexier, iterative innovation has contributed a great deal into making operations easier, safer, and shorter. Disruptive innovations come about every 50 years of thereabouts. Iterative innovations are nearly daily events.

The Innovation Team

It is extremely rare that a major disruptive innovation will be created by a single individual. While team science is the story of the day, history tells us that it is often two or more individuals who are most important in creating important innovations. The credit for innovation is usually given to the idea person, the individual who sees the possibility, who has the imagination, and who is often sufficiently charismatic to "sell" the idea to one or more people who can develop it. This brings us to the important second member of the team, usually an engineer, who is able to turn the idea into a product. Such teams are well known to us: Steve Jobs envisioned the home computer, and Wozniak built it in his garage; Albert Starr and Thomas Fogarty envisioned heart valves and catheters to remove blood clots both of which were developed into products by a brilliant engineer by the name of Lowell Edwards; Charlie Dotter dreamed of dilating arteries of plastic catheters and William Cook built those catheters for Dr. Dotter. While two individuals seem to be the minimum necessary to get started, it takes a village to finish an innovation. One of the most valuable but often overlooked members of an innovative team are the critics, who point out flaws in thinking, flaws in design, or flaws in application. These individuals are capable of keeping an innovative team on track and help prevent the wasting of valuable time and resources. Innovation needs market analysts, to determine whether there is a niche for the innovation. Financiers come in many forms, from federal granting agencies to foundations, to angel investors, and to venture capitalists. There is no successful innovation that is developed without adequate funding. Any device worth making is worth patenting a process that involves the investigation of prior patent records and the description of a novel claim. This very specialized field is critical to success in innovation. Then there is the entrepreneur, the CEO of the company that may be developed to launch a new product. If successful there will be a need for sales and marketing individuals and most importantly trainers to demonstrate to surgeons how to use the new product. Faced with such a daunting task, some surgeons find it easier to "pedal" their ideas to existing companies especially those with proficiency and a track record in producing successful products. Other individuals prefer to license their idea for a set period of time to an established company, and others prefer to start a new company around the new product. Each of these methods has reason for recommendation.

Education in Innovation

A question often asked is: Can creativity be taught? In the minds of most creative individuals, the answer to this question is yes. The process of innovation is not simple and instruction is very helpful. Beyond understanding the need for a new product to solve a surgical problem, there are at least five principles for every innovator to grasp [2]. First, the business angle is critical. It is essential that one determine if there is a market for the new product, how big is that market, and what is the price point for entry. Usually if the market is large, one will find individuals interested in investing in a good idea. However, it is still most important to identify areas where investors or granting agencies are interested. The second element is understanding whether there is new intellectual property in the idea. If the innovation is "obvious," it cannot be patented. This is usually not a great barrier because most solutions that are "obvious" are roads that have longed been explored by others in the areas where it is virtually impossible to protect a new idea. The next question along these lines is the saturation of the market in this area. If you are planning on adding another line to the highway, it is probably not worth the money spent. An innovator looks for open space where there is room to move in several directions adding additional claims to the patent as the space is occupied. Fourth, finding a clever engineer is a necessity. Engineering is a vast field with multiple specialties within it. A good general engineer will probably need to identify subcontractors to help with the design of any sophisticated product. Therefore, it is necessary to identify a senior, well-connected engineer who knows where to go for help. Lastly, education on how to pitch the product is very important. Certainly one can learn a lot by watching "Shark Tank," but in medicine the product pitch is somewhat different generally appealing to a slightly higher level of talent and sophistication.

The Drive to Innovate

There are certain surgeons who are always innovating and others who do not. The drive to innovate is born out of scientific curiosity but with a very practical bent. It is not the financial rewards that drive creative processes. It is not the drive for a royalty, a new company, or a new car that drives surgeons to stay up late and work weekends on a new product. The drive to innovate is generally a drive to make things work better (iterative innovation) or is the desire to bring new developments to fix an old problem (disruptive innovation). One strong theme is that of mastery. We innovate because we desire to improve performance, of a device, of a system, or of ourselves to benefit the patient. At times it is the desire to fix that which is perceived to be broken, a belief that there must be a better way. Innovation engages the imagination and creativity and allows the surgeon expression in way that are seldom possible in the operation room. To quote Daniel Pink, "In innovation we engage our desire for autonomy, mastery, and purpose the three highest motivators of all human behavior" [3].

Conclusion

The history of surgery is the history of innovation. When one creates a list of leaders in surgery from Halsted to DeBakey to Berci, the theme is innovation and a single-minded pursuit to improve performance in surgery for the benefit of the patient. To be a successful innovator, one must possess imagination combined with a laser sharp focus on the problem at hand. Innovation requires team building, physicians, engineers, and entrepreneurs. Rarely, individuals are successful without tapping into an existing company, or an institutional tech transfer program to assist the innovator. To be a successful innovator, one must have the passion to make a difference.

References

1. Christensen C. The innovators prescription: a disruptive solution for health care. New York: McGraw-Hill; 2008.
2. Riskin D, Longaker M, Gertner M, Krummel T. Innovation in surgery: a historical perspective. Ann Surg. 2006;244:686–93.
3. Pink D. Drive: the surprising truth about what motivates us. New York: Penguin Group; 2011.

2. Examples of Innovation by Surgeons: Percutaneous Endoscopic Gastrostomy and Its Ethical Implications

Jeffrey L. Ponsky and John H. Rodriguez

It has been nearly four decades since the first performance of a percutaneous endoscopic gastrostomy [1, 2]. Small children with severe neurological impairment were first to receive this intervention and, as it happened, were benefitted by it [3]. The success of these early cases led to performance of the technique in adults and then to expansion of the indications for the procedure. Only later was laboratory investigation of the issues of tract formation and tube materials undertaken. There were no Institutional Review Boards (IRBs) at that time, and innovative therapy was quickly transformed into standard practice. Several versions of the method were developed, but ironically, over the following decades, the technique has remained much the same. However, the frequency with which PEG is performed has mushroomed, making it one of the most frequent indications for upper GI endoscopy [4]. Examination of the indications for PEG placement and the ethical implications that have accompanied this innovation may be worth examination.

Indications for PEG

The most frequent indication for performance of PEG is the need to provide feedings to patients unable to ingest adequate nutrition [2, 4]. Patients with neurological compromise or oro-pharyngeal tumors are the most commonly seen, although others including those with failure to thrive and the need for supplemental nutrition are also candidates [4, 5].

© Springer International Publishing Switzerland 2016
S.C. Stain et al. (eds.), *The SAGES Manual Ethics of Surgical Innovation*, DOI 10.1007/978-3-319-27663-2_2

The ethical dilemma arises from the question of what role feeding plays in the long-term outcome of the patient [6].

Clearly, patients with both traumatic brain injury (TBI) and a good prognosis for recovery will be well served by PEG. After weeks or months, it is expected that they will recover and resume eating. Other TBI patients with an inability to eat but the likelihood of recovery of some cognitive function are also good candidates [7]. In contrast, the use of PEG for long-term feeding in patients with little hope of recovery is a point of great controversy.

Patients with severe dementia, the elderly with unrecoverable strokes, and those in persistent vegetative states are frequently referred to the surgeon for PEG placement, yet the question of what the procedure offers them is debated [5]. Clearly, the nursing care of a neurologically devastated patient is greatly facilitated by PEG. Indeed, most long-term nursing facilities will require a PEG rather than a naso-enteric tube for feeding and medication administration. However, the provision of long-term feeding in such cases may prolong the duration of suffering, add expense, and prove a burden to a family [8]. Once PEG feeding is commenced, it may be difficult to terminate. In addition, complications arising from the PEG, such as peri-tubal leakage, skin excoriation, and tube dysfunction, may occasionally become a major focus of care in an otherwise hopeless case. Inpatient doctors may ask for a PEG just to facilitate transfer of an apparently hopeless patient from an acute care hospital to a long-term nursing home. The consideration and discussion of what such a decision will do for and to the patient and the family is quite often minimal, and that should not be the case.

The use of PEG for temporary feeding or supplemental nutrition when recovery is likely is unquestionably valuable and appropriate. In cases where the potential for recovery is uncertain but possible, again PEG placement may be appropriate. It is the irretrievable cases where the ethical questions arise. One way to address this issue is to request that all intercurrent problems such as pneumonia, sepsis, and multiorgan failure be corrected prior to placement of the PEG and that nutrition be provided by a naso-enteric tube until the time that PEG is agreed upon.

Patients with oro-pharyngeal tumors often benefit from PEG placement early in their course to provide nutrition while they undergo radiation, chemotherapy, and surgery. In most cases, the PEG is removed after successful treatment as they resume the ability to take oral feedings [9]. This is very gratifying. In cases where the oro-pharyngeal tumor returns and limits oral intake, the PEG may be placed again to permit the terminally ill patient to function better for the time that they have remaining. Again, this use of PEG is quite gratifying as it permits the patient to go about his or her daily activities without the stigma of an indwelling nasal tube. Interestingly, some head and neck surgeons believe that patients who are able to take oral feedings during their therapeutic course, rather than exclusively PEG feedings, may have a lower incidence of esophageal stricture formation after radiation therapy [5].

The use of PEG for gastric decompression in patients with complicated bowel obstruction or carcinomatosis has proven a valuable adjunct to patient care [10]. Rather than extending life in patients with complicated intraabdominal malignancy, the PEG serves merely as a vent to the stomach, and it may reduce gastric distention and emesis. It should be remembered that although the PEG serves as a "vent" in these cases, it may not totally empty the stomach and thus aspiration may still occur.

In patients with recalcitrant bowel obstruction, the performance of a PEG may permit long-term gastric decompression and avoidance of a nasogastric tube, while nutrition is provided by parenteral means. When gastric atony is the diagnosis, some patients benefit from PEG for decompression when it is offered in concert with direct jejunostomy for feeding. Jejunal extension tubes in conjunction with PEG are rarely functional for long, and they are often a constant source of frustration for both the doctor and the patient. Repeated placement of jejunal extension tubes is costly and usually ineffective [11]. When jejunal feedings are anticipated to be necessary for the long term, a direct jejunostomy by means of endoscopy or surgery is a better solution.

Conclusion

The development of the first PEG in 1979 was the result of need, vision, and ingenuity—there was no university or industry sponsor, no mechanical testing or preclinical study, and no clinical trial. Such a progression would be unlikely to occur today. In spite of its humble development, PEG has become one of the most common endoscopic procedures performed today. With the widespread adoption of this innovation have come a host of ethical considerations. Indications for PEG placement vary, and there should be strong consideration of the true benefit of this procedure and its overall impact on the quality of life and prognosis of the patient.

References

1. Ponsky JL. The development of PEG: how it was. J Interv Gastroenterol. 2011; 1(2):88–9.
2. Gauderer MW, Ponsky JL, Izant RJ. Gastrostomy without laparotomy: a percutaneous endoscopic technique. J Pediatr Surg. 1980;15:872–5 [PMID: 6780678].
3. Ponsky JL, Gauderer MW. Percutaneous endoscopic gastrostomy: a nonoperative technique for feeding gastrostomy. Gastrointest Endosc. 1981;27(1):9–11 [PMID: 6783471].
4. Rahnemai-Azar AA, Rahnemaiazar AA, Naghshizadian R, Kurtz A, Farkas DT. Percutaneous endoscopic gastrostomy: indications, technique, complications and management. World J Gastroenterol. 2014;20(24):7739–51 [PMID:24976711].
5. Mekhail TM, Adelstein DJ, Rybicki LA, Larto MA, Saxton JP, Lavertu P. Enteral nutrition during the treatment of head and neck carcinoma: is a percutaneous endoscopic gastrostomy tube preferable to a nasogastric tube? Cancer. 2001;91:1785–90 [PMID: 11335904].
6. Rimon E, Kagansky N, Levy S. Percutaneous endoscopic gastrostomy; evidence of different prognosis in various patient subgroups. Age Ageing. 2005;34:353–7 [PMID: 15901578].
7. Klodell CT, Carroll M, Carrillo EH, Spain DA. Routine intragastric feeding following traumatic brain injury is safe and well tolerated. Am J Surg. 2000;179(3):168–71 [PMID:10827311].
8. Wolfsen HC, Kozarek RA, Ball TJ, Patterson DJ, Botoman VA, Ryan JA. Long-term survival in patients undergoing percutaneous endoscopic gastrostomy and jejunostomy. Am J Gastroenterol. 1990;85:1120–2 [PMID: 2117851].
9. Nugent B, Lewis S, O'Sullivan JM. Enteral feeding methods for nutritional management in patients with head and neck cancers being treated with radiotherapy and/or chemotherapy. Cochrane Database Syst Rev. 2013;1, CD007904 [PMID: 23440820].
10. Kawata N, Kakushima N, Tanaka M, Sawai H, Imai K, Hagiwara T, Takao T, Hotta K, Yamaguchi Y, Takizawa K, Matsubayashi H, Ono H. Percutaneous endoscopic gastrostomy for decompression of malignant bowel obstruction. Dig Endosc. 2014; 26(2):208–13 [PMID: 23772988].
11. Zopf Y, Rabe C, Bruckmoser T, Maiss J, Hahn EG, Schwab D. Percutaneous endoscopic jejunostomy and jejunal extension tube through percutaneous endoscopic gastrostomy: a retrospective analysis of success, complications and outcome. Digestion. 2009;79(2):92–7 [PMID: 19279384].

3. Examples of Innovation by Surgeons: Endoscopic Variceal Ligation

Gregory Van Stiegmann

Major changes in treatment of patients with bleeding esophageal varices occurred during the decade of the 1980s. Dissatisfaction with short- and long-term results of shunt operations led to the re-emergence of endoscopic sclerotherapy. This technique, initially described in the 1930s, was performed by surgeons in an operating room using rigid endoscopes and general anesthesia [1]. Sclerotherapy using flexible fiber-optic endoscopes, performed in an endoscopy suite or intensive care unit under conscious sedation, rapidly replaced the older method. Flexible endoscopic sclerotherapy was widely adopted as an inexpensive, simple to perform, and relatively effective treatment for control of variceal hemorrhage. Elective repeated sclerotherapy treatments, aimed at obliterating varices from the distal esophagus, decreased the incidence of recurrent bleeding. As experience with endoscopic sclerotherapy for esophageal varices increased, it became apparent that injection of caustic sclerosants into the distal esophagus was associated with a substantial risk of both local and systemic complications. Esophageal stricture, bleeding from sclerotherapy-induced ulcerations, chemical necrosis with perforation of the esophageal wall, and sclerosant-induced respiratory distress became recognized accompaniments of injection therapy. At a time when the mortality associated with acute variceal bleeding was as high as 50 %, these shortcomings of injection sclerotherapy seemed relatively inconsequential [2].

Elastic band ligation for the treatment of bleeding from hemorrhoids was first described in the 1960s [3]. Prior to the introduction of this technique, injection sclerotherapy performed via an anoscope, or surgery, were the two mainstays for treating this common problem. Elastic

© Springer International Publishing Switzerland 2016
S.C. Stain et al. (eds.), *The SAGES Manual Ethics
of Surgical Innovation*, DOI 10.1007/978-3-319-27663-2_3

band ligation for treating hemorrhoids was widely accepted and employed in the United States by the 1980s. Surgical treatment became reserved for the few patients that failed band ligation or those with advanced hemorrhoid disease. Elastic band ligation was subsequently found superior to sclerotherapy for treatment of hemorrhoids and required fewer treatment sessions [4].

During the late 1970s and early 1980s, I had the privilege of working as a senior registrar and subsequently as a flexible endoscopic fellow with Professors John Terblanche and Philippus (Flip) Bornman at the Groote Schuur Hospital in the Department of Surgery at the University of Cape Town. Groote Schuur, at that time, was the epicenter for a renaissance of endoscopic sclerotherapy treatment for bleeding esophageal varices. Patients were treated under general anesthesia in the operating room using rigid esophagoscopes and long injection needles. Results were encouraging and few patients required surgical salvage [5]. The shift from operative to endoscopic treatment of bleeding esophageal varices had begun.

I returned to Denver and the Department of Surgery at the University of Colorado with substantial experience in rigid endoscopic sclerotherapy as well as diagnostic and therapeutic (such as existed then) flexible endoscopy skills. As the most junior member of the surgical faculty, my clinic assignments consisted largely of cases my senior colleagues had little interest in. Among these were a number of patients with symptomatic hemorrhoid problems, most of whom were successfully managed using the McGivney elastic band ligating device (Miltex Instrument Co., Lake Success, NY). This technique is performed via an anoscope using a clamp to grasp the hemorrhoid and pull it into the ligating chamber after which the elastic band is ejected to ensnare the captured hemorrhoid. As my experience with elastic band ligation grew, I came to appreciate the simplicity, reproducibility, and effectiveness of this treatment. I wondered if there were other potential applications in the gastrointestinal tract for elastic band ligation.

The Initial Concept

The only similarity between ano-rectal hemorrhoids and esophageal varices is their proclivity to cause problems by bleeding. Anatomically, hemorrhoids are cavernous vascular tissues as compared with esophageal varices that are large thin-walled collateral veins located in the submucosa of the distal esophagus. Could the latter be as effectively treated as the former using elastic band ligation? My initial concept for elastic band ligation of esophageal varices consisted of an elongated McGiveny type ligation device that would be passed through a rigid esophagoscope. The varix would be grasped with a long clamp and drawn into the ligation chamber followed by ejection of the elastic band around the varix to be ensnared. This concept turned out to be little more than a thought exercise. There was no interest whatsoever in making a prototype device for this purpose among any of the manufacturers with whom I discussed the concept. The main reason there was no interest was widespread recognition that rigid endoscopy was rapidly being displaced by flexible endoscopy, including flexible endoscopic sclerotherapy for bleeding esophageal varices.

The Subsequent Concept

Months later, I was supervising a resident performing a flexible sigmoidoscopy. The resident proudly proclaimed he had found an unusual polyp. I peered through the teaching head (video endoscopy was barely introduced then) and advised him that he was the cause of the "polyp." I was demonstrating to the resident how a "suction polyp" is created by inadvertently aspirating mucosa into the biopsy channel, when suddenly a light bulb flashed on. If one had an open ended cylinder mounted on the distal end of a flexible endoscope, could one create a large "suction polyp" that would be amenable to ligation with an elastic band? Suction was the potential key to making elastic band ligation with flexible endoscopes a reality and was a decidedly more elegant solution than grasping a fragile thin-walled vein with a clamp and then pulling on it.

The next step was to get a prototype device built in order to prove the concept was mechanically viable. I was reluctant to disclose many details of what I envisioned the ligating instrument would look like or how it would function, if it functioned at all. I first consulted Mr. Warren Bielke who was national sales director for Pentax Precision Instruments (Orangeburg, NY). I told him I had a concept that I outlined in sketchy detail. I needed a flexible endoscope with the old style screw on (threaded) end cap that could be used to attach an instrument in order to do some animal studies. Pentax Precision Instruments would have first rights to commercialize the device if the concept worked and they were interested. He generously loaned the equipment and we were over the first hurdle.

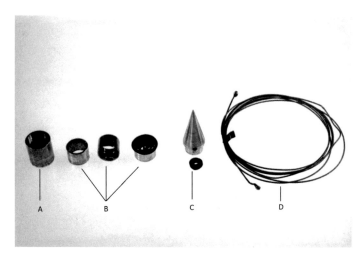

Fig. 3.1. Components of the original endoscopic ligating device prototype. The large cylinder (**a**) attached to the endoscope via screw threads. The inner (banding) cylinders (**b**) were preloaded with elastic bands using the loading cone (**c**). The trip wire (**d**) passed through the biopsy channel and attached to the inner cylinder. All components were stainless steel. (From Stiegmann et al. [6], with permission from Elsevier).

The second hurdle was designing and building a prototype device. The estimate for creation of a medical grade reusable instrument that could be screw mounted to a flexible endoscope was 5000 dollars. An unexpected opportunity to consult for a start-up company that was developing a flexible vascular endoscope resulted in the funds needed to engineer and manufacture one device. The specifications for the original device were driven by the diameter of the endoscope since mounting of the external housing cylinder to the endoscope was to be accomplished using a threaded connection. A shorter, smaller diameter inner (ligating) cylinder, over which an elastic "O" ring was stretched, fit inside the housing cylinder and was connected by cable running through the biopsy channel of the endoscope to the operator. The final component was the loading cone that fit into the inner (ligating) cylinder and facilitated stretching the elastic "O" ring in place over the ligating cylinder. (Figs. 3.1, 3.2, 3.3, and 3.4)

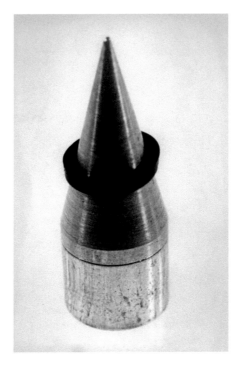

Fig. 3.2. The "O" ring is being loaded onto the banding cylinder using the loading cone. (From Stiegmann et al. [6], with permission from Elsevier).

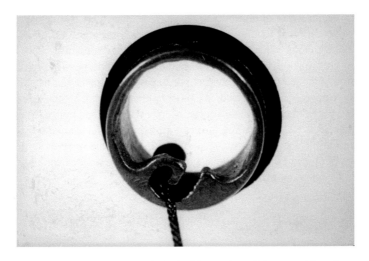

Fig. 3.3. The trip wire, passed via the biopsy channel, is secured into the notch of the inner (ligating) cylinder. Note the elastic "O" ring mounted on the distal end of the ligating cylinder. (From Stiegmann et al. [6], with permission from Elsevier).

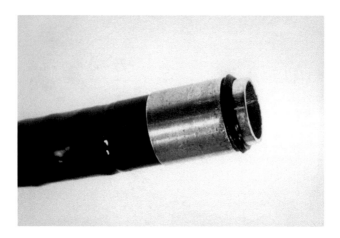

Fig. 3.4. The assembled ligating device. The ligating cylinder with loaded "O" ring is positioned inside the housing cylinder that is attached by screw thread mount to the endoscope. The trip wire runs via the endoscope biopsy channel and exits at the biopsy channel entrance. (From Stiegmann et al. [6], with permission from Elsevier).

Proving the Concept I

Once manufacture of a prototype device appeared likely, we devised a plan to determine if ligating tissue inside the gastrointestinal tract with elastic bands, using a flexible endoscope, could be reproducibly accomplished. This and subsequent animal studies were made possible by a grant from the Veterans Administration that was obtained just as the original prototype was delivered. We quickly confirmed, in a small preliminary study done in normal canines, exactly what we had hoped. The procedure was relatively simple to perform using an endoscopic overtube passed into the esophagus, resulted in no immediate or short-term adverse effects we could recognize and was easy to reproduce multiple times in the same animal [6]. We were elated.

Protecting the Concept

Soon after being convinced that elastic band ligation could be reproducibly performed in animals, I sought intellectual property protection in conjunction with the technology transfer office at the University of

Colorado. The practice of that office, at the time, was to proceed with a preliminary patent filing only, until there was certainty the idea would be commercialized. This stance raised the ante for completion of animal studies, initiation of clinical trials, and finding a manufacturer interested in taking the new method to market. We discussed the advisability of publishing results, in the context of intellectual property protection, prior to obtaining a completed patent. I was erroneously advised that the preliminary filing was adequately protective. That advice was correct if one were only concerned about rights in the United States. I was sorry to learn later that our early publications had effectively eliminated the opportunity to obtain international patent protection.

Proving the Concept II

The next experimental step was a study aimed at examining the clinical and histologic effects of endoscopic ligation on esophageal varices in a portal hypertensive animal model. This work took nearly a year to complete since the dogs had to undergo a laparotomy for creation of the portal hypertension inducing venous anatomy after which several months were required for the esophageal varices that developed to enlarge and mature [7]. Animals were treated with elastic band ligation, followed by repeat endoscopy, and then sacrificed at varying intervals. Detailed histological analysis of the elastic band ligation sites was performed. This study demonstrated, in a portal hypertensive canine model, that the series of local events that occurred in treated tissues included: ischemic necrosis, acute inflammation, shallow ulcer formation, and subsequent healing with re-epithelialization of the ulcer by 14–21 days. Varices in the submucosa were obliterated by a process of dense scar formation. The underlying muscular wall of the esophagus was unaffected. More importantly, throughout this study we observed no adverse clinically apparent events in any of the treated animals [8].

As the course of this animal study progressed, it became apparent that the technique was safe to perform and, from my perspective, was ready to move into human clinical trials. At the time, our Gastroenterology colleagues were rapidly and successfully adopting flexible endoscopic sclerotherapy for treatment of their patients with bleeding esophageal varices. It was clear if we were to move forward clinically in an optimal fashion, a respected Gastroenterologist-Endoscopist needed to join the team. To that end, I invited Dr. John Goff to the animal laboratory one day as we were performing endoscopic ligation on a dog. I had worked with Dr. Goff clinically for several years, and we had a solid relationship in taking care of patients with complex gastrointestinal and biliary problems. I showed him our sole endoscopic ligating instrument, explained how we were using it, and jokingly told him that "I wasn't sure a Gastroenterologist could figure out how to make this work." Of course, as expected, he succeeded on the first try and immediately sensed we were on to something promising. After reviewing the data that had accumulated thus far in the study, he was more convinced. When asked if he had interest in joining forces for a clinical trial, the answer was a resounding yes. That marked the beginning of a productive collaboration as we geared up to determine how endoscopic ligation compared with endoscopic sclerotherapy in patients.

Preliminary Clinical Experience

Institutional Review Board approval of the initial human pilot study was based on the findings from our experimental animal studies and substantial literature confirming the safety and efficacy of treating hemorrhoids using elastic band ligation. Our first patient was a very nice lady who worked as an AT&T telephone operator. She had portal hypertension from chronic hepatitis and was admitted with a variceal bleed. Her band ligation treatment was accomplished without problem. Humans with portal hypertension and variceal bleeding tend to have large varices in contrast to the relatively small ones that developed in our canine model. This made treatment in patients (at least the first treatment session) easier than in the canine since there was more tissue to aspirate into the device and ligate. She was kind enough to allow us to do several diagnostic endoscopies while we observed her in hospital. We observed (and subsequently confirmed in additional patients) essentially the same progression of events at ligated sites in patients that we found in the canines. The initial clinical results bolstered our confidence and set the stage for moving forward with more definitive trials [9]. Before taking the next step, however, we needed to find someone to manufacture the ligating device. All of our work to this point had been done with the original prototype. We realized how tenuous continued progress was when one day, while being washed after use, a key component of the ligating device disappeared down the sink's drain. The plumber was impressed with the number of people interested in his work that afternoon. He successfully retrieved the part.

Commercialization

Numerous representatives and delegations from flexible endoscope manufacturers and endoscopic accessory companies came to Denver. Live demonstrations, endoscopic video tapes, and experimental as well as clinical results were offered up for them. All asked for some time to think about committing to manufacture and market this new treatment concept, including our original supporters at Pentax Precision Instruments. We gained additional experience with clinical use, prepared more presentations for the spring meetings, and became more confident that band ligation was superior to sclerotherapy. Still, no one stepped forward.

At Digestive Disease Week (DDW), I was carrying around a video that demonstrated elastic band ligation in several patients with bleeding varices. Anyone interested was welcome to have a look. I spotted Warren Bielke at the Pentax exhibit and asked him if he had interest in what we had been able to accomplish with the endoscope he had lent us. I plugged the video tape into a relatively public video cassette player and pushed the play button. Several minutes into the showing a well-dressed Japanese man appeared and joined us. I was introduced to Mr Katsumi Oneda, the president of Pentax Precision Instruments. He almost immediately told Mr Bielke to please shut off the video and retrieve the tape from the machine. I was temporarily shocked. Mr Oneda then said "We should not be viewing this in public. Please bring the tape into our private office." In private, we reviewed the video tape, I explained our experimental and clinical results, and Mr. Bielke explained the role Pentax Precision Instruments had played in developing this method. With no hesitation, Mr Oneda simply said: "We want it." The game was on.

During further discussions at DDW and subsequently, I outlined steps I believed necessary to properly test and debut this new treatment in an ideal manner. The first, of course, was manufacturing the device itself. Working with engineers at a Rhode Island injection molding company, the initial production device came to life with only minor design changes that included a "slip on" method of securing the device to the new generations of flexible endoscopes that did not have threaded screw tips on the distal end of the endoscope. The production design was manufactured from molded plastic as a single-use instrument. How to make the trip wire, which in the original prototype was a braided stainless steel cable, was another question. The owner of the company had an idea. He took me out to his car and opened the trunk to reveal a collection of deep sea fishing equipment including several rolls of high-test monofilament fishing line. We settled on the 250 lb. test line and that remains the material in use today.

Once production of devices began, I lobbied for a multicenter prospective randomized trial that would compare endoscopic ligation with endoscopic sclerotherapy. The trial would be conducted by individuals with recognized experience in endoscopic sclerotherapy at five or six centers in the United States. There was immediate question of the cost of such a trial. I believed there was enough interest from highly qualified individuals that if Pentax Precision Instruments could provide the ligating devices and an endoscope for six centers, the local principle investigators would be anxious to put the new method to the test, be an author on a high-quality randomized controlled trial, and have access to the non-Food and Drug Administration (FDA) approved ligating device well ahead of the general endoscopic public. That logic was accepted and planning for a multicenter trial began in earnest.

Over the ensuing months, I learned that Mr. Oneda and his associates Messrs. Lewis Pell and Warren Bielke were highly regarded in the medical device business for developing new devices into successful products using start-up companies that were financed with venture capital. Several months later I found myself in Orangeburg New York presenting the endoscopic ligation concept and the entire context of treatment for bleeding esophageal varices to an assembled group of nonmedical venture capitalists. Several other creative new device ideas were packaged up along with endoscopic ligation and a new company called VascuCare was formed. Some months thereafter, the marketing rights for endoscopic ligation were acquired by Bard Interventional Products, a flexible endoscopy focused division of the C. R. Bard Company.

Working with Bard Interventional engineers, the design of the endoscopic ligating device was optimized and considerations for packaging and the quantities of preloaded elastic "O" rings that should be included in each kit were addressed. The main issue for Bard Interventional, however, was obtaining FDA approval in order to begin marketing the ligating device. Options included an "Investigational Device Exemption" pathway that could take several years to complete, or the 510-K pathway of demonstrating substantial equivalence to devices currently marketed. The latter was much shorter. I suggested to the team at Bard that endoscopic band ligation used for treatment of hemorrhoids was identical to elastic band ligation for hemorrhoids performed using other devices currently on the market. I further suggested that if endoscopists wanted to use band ligation for "off label" purposes, such as treating esophageal varices, that was a medical decision left to their discretion. After about a year, the Bard endoscopic ligating device came to market approved by the FDA as a hemorrhoid treatment method. Few people using it at the time bothered to read the package inserts.

Everything was coming together. The patent filing was completed and eventually approved. Leadership at Bard Interventional was passed to Mr. David Chazanovitz who was a friend and innovative business leader. The prospective randomized multicenter trial was running smoothly and data acquisition was nearly complete. We knew, from an interim analysis, that there were strong trends favoring endoscopic ligation in almost all of the variables measured. Dr. Goff's and my biggest problem was trying to accommodate all of the invitations we received to speak on the subject. Additional data began to emerge from other institutions both in North America and abroad that confirmed our initial observations and clinical results. Then, one afternoon, I received a telephone call. The endoscopic ligating device was being removed from the market.

The Bard Cardiovascular division had apparently modified the design of one of its cardiac catheters and had not made corresponding changes in the package insert or notified the FDA of the minor changes. This was a major issue for the FDA and resulted in all C. R. Bard divisions scouring their product package inserts to make certain everything was in order. When the endoscopic ligating device package insert was reviewed, it was realized that almost all of the devices sold were being used to treat bleeding esophageal varices, an indication for which the device had not been approved by the FDA. This was a bit of a crisis; however, the timing could not have been better. We had just received word that results from our multicenter trial comparing endoscopic ligation with sclerotherapy had been accepted for publication by the New England Journal of Medicine [10]. Our trial results and additional clinical data generated by others provided solid evidence that elastic bland ligation treatment for bleeding varices was safer, more effective, and more efficient than endoscopic sclerotherapy. These data were submitted to the FDA and, ironically, resulted in the first medical device approved for a specific clinical indication based on prospective randomized clinical trial data.

Epilogue

Endoscopic elastic bland ligation has been the endoscopic treatment of choice for bleeding esophageal varices for 20 years. Development of a multifire device by Saeed, one of our multicenter study principle investigators, greatly simplified and accelerated acceptance of the method [11]. Numerous prospective, randomized studies have reconfirmed our original findings as has meta-analysis of these data [12].

It is unclear if endoscopic elastic band ligation would have been developed if the regulatory milieu of the 1980s were similar to that of today. The complex and costly restrictions faced by today's surgical innovators were imposed with the best intentions. The consequences, however, discourage creativity and diminish progress.

References

1. Craafoord C, Frenkner P. New surgical treatment of varicose veins of the esophagus. Acta Otolaryngol (Stockh). 1939;27:422.
2. Chalasani N, Kahi C, Francois F, Pinto A, Marathe A, Bini EJ, et al. Improved patient survival after acute variceal bleeding: a multicenter, cohort study. Am J Gastroenterol. 2003;98(3):653–9.
3. Barron J. Office ligation of internal hemorrhoids. Am J Surg. 1963;105:563–70.
4. MacRae HM, McLeod RS. Comparison of hemorrhoidal treatments: a meta-analysis. Can J Surg. 1997;40(1):14–7.
5. Terblanche J, Yakoob HI, Bornman PC, Stiegmann GV, Bane R, Jonker M, et al. Acute bleeding varices: a five-year prospective evaluation of tamponade and sclerotherapy. Ann Surg. 1981;194(4):521–30.
6. Stiegmann GV, Cambre T, Sun JH. A new elastic band ligating device. Gastrointest Endosc. 1986;32(3):230–3.
7. Jensen DM, Machicado GA, Tapia JI, Kauffman G, Franco P, Beilin D. A reproducible canine model of esophageal varices. Gastroenterology. 1983;84(3):573–9.
8. Stiegmann GV, Sun JH, Hammond W. Results of experimental endoscopic esophageal varix ligation. Am Surg. 1988;54:105–8.
9. Van Stiegmann G, Goff JS. Endoscopic esophageal varix ligation: preliminary clinical experience. Gastrointest Endosc. 1988;34(2):113–7.
10. Stiegmann GV, Goff JS, Michaletz-Onody PA, Korula J, Lieberman D, Saeed ZA, et al. Endoscopic sclerotherapy as compared with endoscopic ligation for bleeding esophageal varices. N Engl J Med. 1992;326(23):1527–32.
11. Saeed ZA. The Saeed Six-Shooter: a prospective study of a new endoscopic multiple rubber-band ligator for the treatment of varices. Endoscopy. 1996;28(7):559–64.
12. Laine L, Cook D. Endoscopic ligation compared with sclerotherapy for treatment of esophageal variceal bleeding. A meta-analysis. Ann Intern Med. 1995;123(4):280–7.

4. Examples of Surgical Innovation by Surgeons: Natural Orifice Transluminal Endoscopic Surgery

Peter Nau and David W. Rattner

Whether considering the practice of bloodletting or the concept of balancing of the four humors, the practice of medicine has undergone countless innovations throughout its history. As early as 1805, Phillip Bozzini was using his leather-covered, vase-shaped Lichtleiter to complete cystoscopies using a canine model [1]. Unfortunately, during a review by the Medical Faculty of Vienna, his invention was dismissed merely as a magic lantern [2]. Following this critique, both his career and invention fell into obscurity, never to recover from the myopic review by his contemporaries. His critics clearly lacked the foresight to realize his invention would become the foundation of cystoscopy, one of the most common procedures performed in modern urology. Notwithstanding the severity of the Lichtleiter's rebuke, the introduction of novel approaches to the treatment of common surgical pathology should be subject to the scrutiny of a rigorous review process. When new devices or procedures are introduced, it is the ethical obligation of surgeons to ensure that a patient's safety comes first. Nowhere is this more important than with the concept of natural orifice transluminal endoscopic surgery (NOTES). Regardless of its minimally invasive qualities, NOTES is a technique whose safety and efficacy must be vetted in a transparent manner prior to its widespread promotion.

© Springer International Publishing Switzerland 2016   25
S.C. Stain et al. (eds.), *The SAGES Manual Ethics
of Surgical Innovation*, DOI 10.1007/978-3-319-27663-2_4

Defining the Problem

The practice of drug development and commercialization is a painstaking process during which the new drug is evaluated at multiple stages for both safety and efficacy. The Food and Drug Administration (FDA) is intimately involved in this progression. Likewise, the FDA must approve new surgical devices after determining that they are safe and effective for the indications specified in the manufacturer's application. Since the FDA is not empowered to regulate novel surgical procedures, it can only influence their introduction by deeming the use of essential devices as high risk and raising the bar for these devices regulatory clearance. While there are clear federal guidelines for research involving human subjects, there is little guidance regarding the introduction of new techniques utilized in the operating room [3, 4]. Nowhere was this better illustrated than with the mass rollout of the laparoscopic cholecystectomy in the early 1990s. Responding principally to market forces, consumer demand, and a push from the medical device industry, many surgeons completed cursory weekend courses and then performed laparoscopic cholecystectomies on their patients, learning on the job as they acquired experience with this new technique. The result was significant increase in the incidence of common bile duct injury when compared to an open approach [5, 6]. With this fact in mind, the early leaders in the field of NOTES drafted what is often referred to as The White Paper [7]. In this document, the authors identified the obstacles that must be overcome for NOTES to achieve widespread success, concluding the document with the statement, "The leadership of SAGES and ASGE is hopeful and enthusiastic about this burgeoning new field and is committed to safely developing and introducing a technology that may benefit patients as the next wave of minimally invasive therapy" (Table 4.1). Critical to this statement is the emphasis placed on safety and the uncertainty of the benefit that NOTES poses to the patient. It is this attention to the ethical transparency in the evolution of the technology that is critical for the success of NOTES.

Ethics and the Evaluation of Notes

One of the most important aspects of the ethical assimilation of techniques using a natural orifice approach is the methods used to evaluate the technology. Historically, surgical innovation was justified by necessity with the alternative being a dire outcome for the patient. In the case

Table 4.1. Potential impediments to the successful implementation of NOTES as identified by the ASGE-SAGES working group.

Access to the peritoneal cavity
Intestinal closure
Prevention of infection
Development of suturing and anastomotic devices
Spatial orientation
Development of a multitasking platform
Management of complications
Physiologic untoward events
Compression syndromes
Training

of NOTES, however, existing elective procedures are usually an acceptable option. Certainly conventional laparoscopic cholecystectomy poses a reasonable morbidity and mortality profile when compared to the transvaginal approach. Given this distinction, it is imperative that the community of surgical endoscopists approach the endorsement of NOTES with a degree of restraint when compared with such groundbreaking discoveries as Lister's concept of antisepsis or DeBakey's use of Dacron grafts for aortic replacement.

Perhaps the most effective method for evaluating the outcomes of the natural orifice approach is through well-designed clinical trials. Historically, this has been accomplished using randomized controlled trials (RCT). With that said, a review of surgical research noted that almost half of the data on innovative surgical techniques are presented in the form of a case series [8]. Unfortunately, there are many limitations to the completion of a RCT in a surgical setting. For one, the execution of a properly powered trial can take a prohibitively long time to the extent that relevance is absent upon completion. Along those same lines, the timing of a trial can be very difficult to pinpoint. If performed too early, a trial has the potential to stymie innovation because of learning curve effects. If addressed to late, a trial may lack clinical relevance [9, 10]. Lastly, the ability to complete a blinded trial or perform a placebo procedure is prohibitively difficult or often unethical. Given this, many investigators have opted for a well-designed, protocol-driven nonrandomized studies. When incorporating prospective design and meticulous data collection, this is an appropriate tool for the evaluation of a new technique.

Unlike much of the history of surgical innovation, which has been characterized by necessity, NOTES has arisen during a time of surgical abundance. An effective and safe approach to most pathology is the standard rather than the exception. Given this, it is important to determine at what level the bar for efficacy and safety must be established. If set to high, the ability to achieve progress is obstructed and too low and patient safety is sacrificed. Perhaps the most ethical approach is to continuously evaluate and re-evaluate NOTES and to remain transparent throughout the process. Using a clinical example, this was the approach used during the assessment of the Angelchik device for the treatment of medically refractory gastroesophageal reflux disease (GERD). In its infancy, clinical trials were undertaken against the gold standard procedure to evaluate for efficacy and safety [11]. Subsequent to these publications, long-term follow-up evaluations were completed [12, 13]. Ultimately, it was noted that this technique was vastly inferior to the gold standard, and the operation has been removed from the treatment algorithm. Perhaps the technology would have been better assessed solely through the use of RCTs. In the absence of this, however, the dedication to maintaining a dialogue on patient welfare and outcomes was the ethical and appropriate course of action. It is this methodology that must be incorporated as NOTES moves forward.

While the ethical evaluation of NOTES from a morbidity and efficacy standpoint is of the utmost importance, it is also imperative that the surgical community defines success and progress. It is only after establishing these expectations that the validity and ethics of utilizing a new technique or approach can be determined. Historically speaking, most innovation has been proposed in an effort to decrease morbidity and mortality. With the recent introduction of natural orifice and single-site surgery, more emphasis has been placed expected improvements on cosmesis and short-term pain scores. Notably, the hypothesis that pain will uniformly decrease with single-site surgery has not consistently born out in the literature [14–16]. Further, a significant increase in the risk of hernia formation was noted in a well-designed, randomized, multicenter, single-blinded trial [17]. Therein lies the crux of novel approaches to classic surgical pathology. Certainly, patient-driven outcomes such as cosmesis and time for convalescence are important. However, it is the ethical responsibility of the surgical community to demonstrate that the proposed benefits are realized and are not outweighed by new complications through thoughtful clinical investigations. Finally, care is being delivered in an ever increasingly cost conscious environment. As such, cost effectiveness is increasingly important in determining whether or not a procedure or medical device will be accepted.

Institutional Review

In 1992, the Lancet published an editorial reviewing the merits of a new antireflux device. In this manuscript, the author states that, "Whenever a new operation or prosthesis is introduced, surgeons must ask three questions: (a) is it safe?; (b) is it more effective, with fewer side effects, than existing treatments?; and (c) is it cost-effective?" [18] Nowhere are these tenets more relevant than with the introduction of NOTES. Natural orifice surgery uses existing devices in novel ways for the completion of previously described procedures. Given that this often does not necessitate the introduction of a new device or medication per se, it typically falls outside of the purview of most hospital regulatory committees. From an ethical perspective, it is vital that all initial introductions of NOTES be done with the oversight of an objective third party such as an Institutional Review Board (IRB).

There is a mistaken tradition in surgery that seemingly small variations in surgical instruments or techniques are merely insignificant modifications of existing procedures than true research, which necessitate formal evaluation by an IRB [4, 19]. It has been suggested that any surgical innovation that seeks to define a new technique, investigates outcomes, or imposes a new set of complications should be submitted for IRB review. Unfortunately, a recent review indicated that the majority of researchers do not request IRB approval despite the endorsement of their procedure as research-based [4]. Many times IRB requirements for documentation and reporting are cumbersome and expensive creating a strong disincentive to request such oversight. Furthermore, not all IRBs hold investigators to the same standards. Some IRBs are perceived by investigators as overzealous, whereas others, perhaps because of institutional priorities to promote clinical trials, are more helpful to the investigators. Irrespective of the local situation, IRB oversight is the most widely accepted way that the process of vetting a new procedure can be ensured. Surgical patients are a potentially vulnerable population in that they are searching for an often extreme answer for a medical ailment. While surgeons may have their patients' best interest in mind, they are subject to biases based on their interpretations of various treatment options as well as financial and academic pressures. Presenting a novel technique such as NOTES for IRB review is an important step in validating the approach. In doing this, the surgeon can ensure the ethical legitimacy of presenting the technique to his or her patient.

Data Collection and Continuing Review

Surgery is unique to the field medicine in that clinical outcomes can take years to mature so as to provide the complete picture of the risk-benefit profile of an operation. A good example of this is the recent experience with the laparoscopic adjustable gastric band. A procedure that was once heralded as the answer to obesity due to its reversibility and safety profile has now been widely abandoned due to inconsistent weight loss and delayed complications necessitating band explantation [20, 21]. This situation is not unique to medicine, emphasizing that the NOTES community must continue to follow this group of patients to evaluate for long-term results.

Prior to the widespread adoption of natural orifice approaches, it is the ethical responsibility of the pioneers in the field to prove that it is a safe and effective alternative to the gold standard. To date, the Natural Orifice Surgery Consortium for Assessment and Research (NOSCAR) has led the way with these efforts. A joint venture between the leaders of the American Society for Gastrointestinal Endoscopy (ASGE) and the Society of American Gastrointestinal and Endoscopic Surgeons, NOSCAR, has consistently advocated for the continuing evaluation of this new technique and actively supports the use of data registries to follow these patients. Furthermore, it is incumbent on individual practitioners endorse appropriate data collection and follow-up in his or her practice. Objective outcomes must be a well-defined and a validated classification system for complications such as the Clavien–Dindo scale used to catalog results (Table 4.2). Additionally, given the patient-centered focus of NOTES, subjective patient assessments must be incorporated into the evaluation process. While morbidity and mortality are easy data points to collect and evaluate, many of the purported benefits of NOTES lie outside these classic metrics. As NOTES moves forward, it will be important to incorporate patient-centric outcomes, cost, and efficacy in the evaluation of the technique.

Table 4.2. Clavien–Dindo classification of surgical complications.

Grade I

Any deviation from the normal postoperative course without the need for pharmacological treatment or surgical, endoscopic, and radiological interventions. Allowed therapeutic regimens are: drugs as antiemetics, antipyretics, analgesics, diuretics, electrolytes, and physiotherapy. This grade also includes wound infections opened at the bedside

Grade II

Requiring pharmacological treatment with drug other than such allowed for grade I complications. Blood transfusions and total parenteral nutrition are included

Grade III

Requiring surgical, endoscopic, or radiological intervention

Grade IIIa: intervention not under general anesthesia

Grade IIIb: intervention under general anesthesia

Grade IV

Life-threatening complication (including CNS complications)* requiring intermediate care or intensive-care unit management

Grade IVa: single-organ dysfunction (including dialysis)

Grade IVb: multiorgan dysfunction

Grade V

Death of a patient

Certainly regular data collection is important to the ethical assessment of NOTES. Perhaps more importantly, it is imperative that there is continuing review of the information with an eye on the ethical validity of the approach. The dissemination of innovative technology exposes both the patient and the surgeon to biases. Many patients will seek out newer technology, assuming that the latest is also the greatest [9, 22]. In the same way, surgeons may lack equipoise about the efficacy and safety profile of a new technique. These facts must be acknowledged and addressed with constant re-evaluation of NOTES. Is this technology being offered for the right reasons to the right people? Has the surgical community placed a premium on innovation rather than patient-centered outcomes? Do the results indicate that this new technique is inferior to the gold standard? In addition to objective surgeon-defined data points, these ethical questions must be continually reassessed during the initial stages of NOTES.

Informed Consent

While the field of NOTES has progressed immeasurably since the first diagnostic peritoneoscopies performed by Kalloo and Kantsevoy, it remains an alternative approach rather than the gold standard [23]. Inherent in this acknowledgment is the ethical dilemma of obtaining truly informed consent. Early in the development of an innovative technique, there is an optimism bias which tends to overestimate the positive effects of a new surgery or instrument [22, 24]. This may lead to the overemphasis of theoretical benefits of a procedure when discussing treatment algorithms with the patient. It is vital that the surgeon and hospital acknowledge these issues so as to remain neutral during these interactions.

The process of obtaining informed consent is fraught with ethical concerns that must be addressed during the physician-patient interaction. In order for a patient to be able to determine which option is most appropriate, he or she must have complete information on the risks, benefits, and alternatives. Inherent in surgical innovation is an inability to disclose all potential outcomes as they are necessarily unknown. Furthermore, the lack of equipoise by the surgeon and the trust placed in physicians by patients generates a situation where informed consent is difficult to achieve. Given these limitations, it is important that the physician not focus on proposed or hypothesized benefits. He or she must instead explicitly outline the experimental technique and review existing data regarding the new procedure [9]. Patients should be informed of the purported indications and informed about the limitations of the exiting follow-up data (if they exist). While unrelated to the technical outcomes of a procedure, this discussion is critical to the ethical introduction of new surgical technology.

A New Training Paradigm

In the drafting of the White Paper, the authors acknowledged the paradigm shift that the introduction of laparoscopy represented. Implicit in this manuscript was the recognition of the impressive growing pains experienced with the reconciliation of laparoscopic skills in a field dominated by open surgery. With that in mind, the White Paper was written to serve as a guide for the responsible development of NOTES [7]. In this way, the authors hoped to prevent the ethical and technical dilemma of how NOTES should progress from single-surgeon case series to widely available approaches to common surgical pathology.

One of the most important concerns with the adoption of surgical innovation is the learning curve inherent in a new technique or surgical instrument. One of the procedures that emerged from the NOTES movement was Per Oral Endoscopic Myotomy (POEM) to treat achalasia. This procedure was initially reported by Inoue in 2009, and he rapidly accumulated experience such that by the time others started performing this procedure he had performed over 100 cases [25]. As POEM was implemented at other medical centers, the question of a learning curve became a very real issue. What's more, many surgeons may not appreciate the length of a learning phase to the incorporation of a new technique until he or she has become extremely facile with the new procedure and can look back and analyze the early cases. This very important ethical issue must be addressed in two distinct phases. Initially, the surgeon should acknowledge to the patient the level of experience he or she has with the procedure. Secondly, all practitioners should adhere to a structured process of acquiring the skills to successfully and safely offer the new technology. In this way, the ethics of the patient interaction are guaranteed.

Returning to the rollout of the laparoscopic cholecystectomy, initial cases were longer and results inferior. However, that is less a reflection of the technique and more of an indictment on the absence of a training paradigm to teach surgeons laparoscopic skills. With that in mind, NOTES proponents have published guidelines for the effective training of future endoscopic surgeons. Al-Akash et al. published a succinct review of the barriers unique to natural orifice surgery including the development of endoscopic skills, the lack of dedicated NOTES simulators, and technical deficiencies such as inferior optics and haptics [26]. Others have authored more specific statements on the steps needed to safely implement POEM into one's treatment algorithm for esophageal dysmotility [27]. As NOTES becomes more prevalent, adherence to these tenets will be essential for maintenance of patient welfare.

Highlighting Success

There have been many attempts to identify procedures for which a NOTES approach is advantageous. Early efforts in a swine model produced reports of diagnostic peritoneoscopies, solid organ resections, and intestinal anastomoses [23, 28, 29]. Similarly, there has been integration of NOTES techniques in human populations for similar procedures [30, 31]. However, nowhere has the approach been as useful as in the treatment of achalasia and rectal cancer. Unlike hybrid transvaginal cholecystectomy, POEM and transanal colorectal resections are not restricted to a female population. Moreover, they have been systematically investigated during their inception. Prior to offering the approach in humans, a NOTES approach to colorectal resections was evaluated in both living swine models and human cadavers [32, 33]. Subsequent to this, the technique was utilized in several small, IRB-approved case series with good success. Similarly, Inoue built upon Pasricha's experience with the submucosal endoscopic myotomy in pigs prior to attempting the humans [34]. Importantly, in each instance, the cases were completed with appropriate third-party review and prospectively controlled patient selection criteria. In the setting of surgical innovation, it is difficult to control for all of the unforeseeable outcomes, presenting an ethical dilemma when featuring a human population. With that said, the aforementioned procedures have proceeded in an ethical and step-wise manner, focusing on patient autonomy and safety.

Conclusion

The history of medicine is replete with innovation, both failed and successful. Natural orifice transluminal endoscopic surgery offers a novel approach to common surgical pathology. As the technique matures, it is important that it remains patient-centric. At every step, surgeons and innovators must ensure that the autonomy and safety of the patient is protected. It is only through this approach that the ethical adoption of NOTES is attainable.

References

1. Morgenstern L. The 200th anniversary of the first endoscope: Philipp Bozzini (1773–1809). Surg Innov. 2005;12(2):105–6.
2. Gorden A. The history and development of endoscopic surgery. London: Saunders; 1993.
3. Office for Human Research Protections maintained by the U.S. Department of Health & Human Services. http://www.hhs.gov/ohrp/index.html

4. Reitsma AM, Moreno JD. Ethical regulations for innovative surgery: the last frontier? J Am Coll Surg. 2002;194(6):792–801.
5. Connor S, Garden OJ. Bile duct injury in the era of laparoscopic cholecystectomy. Br J Surg. 2006;93(2):158–68.
6. Bernard HR, Hartman TW. Complications after laparoscopic cholecystectomy. Am J Surg. 1993;165(4):533–5.
7. Rattner D, Kalloo A, ASGE/SAGES Working Group. ASGE/SAGES Working Group on Natural Orifice Translumenal Endoscopic Surgery. Surg Endosc. 2006;20(2):329–33.
8. Horton R. Surgical research or comic opera: questions, but few answers. Lancet. 1996;347:984–5.
9. Tan VK, Chow PK. An approach to the ethical evaluation of innovative surgical procedures. Ann Acad Med Singapore. 2011;40(1):26–9.
10. Ergina PL, Cook JA, Blazeby JM, et al. Challenges in evaluating surgical innovation. Lancet. 2009;374(9695):1097–104.
11. Kmiot WA, Kirby RM, Akinola D, Temple JG. Prospective randomized trial of Nissen fundoplication and Angelchik prosthesis in the surgical treatment of medically refractory gastro-oesophageal reflux disease. Br J Surg. 1991;78(10):1181–4.
12. Varshney S, Kelly JJ, Branagan G, Somers SS, Kelly JM. Angelchik prosthesis revisited. World J Surg. 2002;26(1):129–33. Epub 2001 Nov 26.
13. Timoney AG, Kelly JM, Welfare MR. The Angelchik antireflux device: a 5-year experience. Ann R Coll Surg Engl. 1990;72(3):185–7.
14. Song T, Cho J, Kim TJ, Kim IR, Hahm TS, Kim BG, Bae DS. Cosmetic outcomes of laparoendoscopic single-site hysterectomy compared with multi-port surgery: randomized controlled trial. J Minim Invasive Gynecol. 2013;20(4):460–7.
15. Song T, Kim MK, Kim ML, Yoon BS, Seong SJ. Would fewer port numbers in laparoscopy produce better cosmesis? Prospective study. J Minim Invasive Gynecol. 2014;21(1):68–73.
16. Saad S, Strassel V, Sauerland S. Randomized clinical trial of single-port, minilaparoscopic and conventional laparoscopic cholecystectomy. Br J Surg. 2013;100(3):339–49.
17. Marks JM, Phillips MS, Tacchino R, et al. Single-incision laparoscopic cholecystectomy is associated with improved cosmesis scoring at the cost of significantly higher hernia rates: 1-year results of a prospective randomized, multicenter, single-blinded trial of traditional multiport laparoscopic cholecystectomy vs single-incision laparoscopic cholecystectomy. J Am Coll Surg. 2013;216(6):1037–47; discussion 1047–8.
18. [No authors listed]. Angelchik revisited: lessons for the introduction of new operations. Lancet. 1992;339(8789):340.
19. Biffl WL, Spain DA, Reitsma AM, et al. Responsible development and application of surgical innovations: a position statement of the Society of University Surgeons. J Am Coll Surg. 2008;206(3):1204–9.
20. Aarts EO, Dogan K, Koehestanie P, Aufenacker TJ, Janssen IM, Berends FJ. Long-term results after laparoscopic adjustable gastric banding: a mean fourteen year follow-up study. Surg Obes Relat Dis. 2014;10(4):633–40.

21. Himpens J, Cadière GB, Bazi M, Vouche M, Cadière B, Dapri G. Long-term outcomes of laparoscopic adjustable gastric banding. Arch Surg. 2011;146(7):802–7.
22. Angelos P. Ethics and surgical innovation: challenges to the professionalism of surgeons. Int J Surg. 2013;11 Suppl 1:S2–5.
23. Kalloo AN, Singh VK, Jagannath SB, Niiyama H, Hill SL, Vaughn CA, Magee CA, Kantsevoy SV. Flexible transgastric peritoneoscopy: a novel approach to diagnostic and therapeutic interventions. Gastrointest Endosc. 2004;60(1):114–7.
24. Johnson J, Rogers W. Innovative surgery: the ethical challenges. J Med Ethics. 2012;38(1):9–12.
25. Inoue H, Minami H, Kobayashi Y, Sato Y, Kaga M, Suzuki M, Satodate H, Odaka N, Itoh H, Kudo S. Peroral endoscopic myotomy (POEM) for esophageal achalasia. Endoscopy. 2010;42:265–71.
26. Al-Akash M, Boyle E, Tanner WA. Training on N.O.T.E.S.: from history we learn. Surg Oncol. 2009;18(2):111–9.
27. Eleftheriadis N, Inoue H, Ikeda H, Onimaru M, Yoshida A, Hosoya T, Maselli R, Kudo SE. Training in peroral endoscopic myotomy (POEM) for esophageal achalasia. Ther Clin Risk Manag. 2012;8:329–42.
28. Park PO, Bergström M, Ikeda K, et al. Experimental studies of transgastric gallbladder surgery: cholecystectomy and cholecystogastric anastomosis. Gastrointest Endosc. 2005;61:601–6.
29. Kantsevoy SV, Jagannath SB, Niiyama H, et al. Endoscopic gastrojejunostomy with survival in a porcine model. Gastrointest Endosc. 2005;62:287–92.
30. Salinas G, Saavedra L, Agurto H, Quispe R, Ramírez E, Grande J, Tamayo J, Sánchez V, Málaga D, Marks JM. Early experience in human hybrid transgastric and transvaginal endoscopic cholecystectomy. Surg Endosc. 2010;24(5):1092–8.
31. Nau P, Anderson J, Happel L, Yuh B, Narula VK, Needleman B, Ellison EC, Melvin WS, Hazey JW. Safe alternative transgastric peritoneal access in humans: NOTES. Surgery. 2011;149(1):147–52.
32. Sylla P, Sohn DK, Cizginer S, Konuk Y, Turner BG, Gee DW, Willingham FF, Hsu M, Mino-Kenudson M, Brugge WR, Rattner DW. Survival study of natural orifice translumenal endoscopic surgery for rectosigmoid resection using transanal endoscopic microsurgery with or without transgastric endoscopic assistance in a swine model. Surg Endosc. 2010;24(8):2022–30.
33. Telem DA, Berger DL, Bordeianou LG, Rattner DW, Sylla P. Update on Transanal NOTES for rectal cancer: transitioning to human trials. Minim Invasive Surg. 2012;2012:287613. doi:10.1155/2012/287613. Epub 2012 May 20.
34. Pasricha PJ, Hawari R, Ahmed I, Chen J, Cotton PB, Hawes RH, Kalloo AN, Kantsevoy SV, Gostout CJ. Submucosal endoscopic esophageal myotomy: a novel experimental approach for the treatment of achalasia. Endoscopy. 2007;39(9):761–4.

5. Managing Conflict of Interest

David W. Easter and Tazo Inui

> *It is not from the benevolence of the butcher, the brewer or the baker that we expect our dinner, but from their regard to their own interest.*
>
> Adam Smith, *Wealth of Nations*, 1776

Surgeons are innovators who manage a variety of conflicts in their everyday practices. We want the best tools possible to allow us to invade our patients' bodies while causing the least physiologic insult and the best chance of success. As such, advances in surgical endoscopy, and the efforts of groups like SAGES, have helped create many ethical conflicts for our practices and our patients—in a good way. Without false egotism, surgeons have always led the way in new device development and have thereby fomented healthy public policy discourse [1–4]. But the relationship between surgeon-innovators and device manufacturers has never been more complicated.

Patients and the media sometimes contribute to the development and acceptance of devices or drugs that are not tested as rigorously as physicians might want, by their push for the "latest and greatest" [5]. They are often willing to accept significant risks—if personal benefit seems likely. A recent survey of morbidly obese patients found that 33 % of pre-op patients would accept a 10 % risk of mortality in order to achieve their desired weight-loss goals [6]. In the context of rising obesity rates, is there any surprise where device companies have focused their recent investments?

This willingness of patients to take significant personal risks occurs regularly in spite of limited available information, including that from underpowered clinical trials. Patients and surgeons want better instruments and better outcomes, but they often must rely on limited data when making choices. The "substantial equivalence" principle behind the FDA

© Springer International Publishing Switzerland 2016
S.C. Stain et al. (eds.), *The SAGES Manual Ethics of Surgical Innovation*, DOI 10.1007/978-3-319-27663-2_5

510k device approval process may contribute to this ethically charged conundrum, wherein some new Class II devices are introduced into our surgical practices without rigorous clinical trials. For example, a 2012 literature review by the FDA of 549 gastric band articles found only a single randomized controlled trial and only 16 case series of more than 20 patients [7]. Only 4 of the 16 case series had a control arm- Ouch. For perspective, approximately 18,000 gastric bands were placed prior to 2008, with surgeons and equipment companies making tidy profits [8].

There exists a complicated relationship between patients, surgeons, and medical device companies, fraught with ethically dueling interests. Companies hope to improve surgical devices and thereby sell clinically and financially successful products. Patients want the best care, which correctly or not, they often confuse with the most recent "advancement" or "discovery," even if there is not good scientific support for it. Surgeons hope to contribute their expertise to the development of clinically beneficial innovations and rightly should do so. Plus, there may be hope by many parties for robust compensation—the invisible hand of capitalism at work.

To help provide "bright lines" that protect both companies and physicians from engaging in scornful or unethical behaviors, a bevy of guidelines have been produced—some with active input from device manufacturers. The Advanced Medical Technology Association (AdvaMed) produced a Code of Ethics on Interactions with Health Care Professionals in 2002 and again in 2009, which included a variety of recommendations [9]. These recommendations, for voluntary implementation, included a limit on gifts to individuals of $100/year, the prohibition of recreational trips, the abolishment of free meals (to the great dismay of residents and program directors), and other limits on areas of perceived impropriety. Regarding reimbursement to a surgeon for his participation in device development, AdvaMed suggested:

> A Company should enter into a royalty arrangement with a Health Care Professional only where the Health Care Professional is expected to make, or has made, a novel, significant, or innovative contribution … [and this should be] appropriately documented.

In other words, "no freebies."

Respectable specialty societies have also published their own conflict of interest disclosure and management guidelines [10–14]. These guidelines usually include the requirement that surgeons involved in device development agree to specific consultant or advisory positions *only if* the need for their expertise is clearly spelled out in advance and in writing.

It is perceived nefarious conflicts of interest, not in keeping with these recommendations, that leads to sensational media headlines, such as (1) "Device Makers Pay High-Volume Spine Surgeons Consulting, Design Fees" (CBS Evening News, May 12, 2014); (2) "FDA Advisers' Financial Ties Not Disclosed" (Wall Street Journal, December 8, 2014); and (3) "Safety Journal Blasts Denham in Conflict of Interest Scandal" (Modern Healthcare, November 26, 2014).

It is a further indication of the growing public and political skepticism of physician impartiality that the Patient Protection and Affordable Care Act of 2010 (Title VI.A.6002) [15] includes a requirement for regular reporting of physician-owned investments in device manufacturers. This reporting also includes the receipt of payments, honoraria, or fees from physician-industry relationships.

Patients, surgeons, and equipment companies are not the only driving forces behind the incorporation of new devices and technologies. Hospitals and practice groups argue that being seen as surgical leaders can make them more visible within their community, adding to market share and fiscal bottom lines. And as the saying goes, *No Money, No Mission.* Have you seen the billboards like "*Our Hospital is the First in Town with DaGizmo Machine*"?

It is in this difficult sociopolitical and legal context that we surgeons need to employ extra careful tactics to disclose and manage any potential, real, or perceived conflicts of interest, especially when participating in surgical innovation. What are these "conflicts of interest," you ask? We offer here several vignettes to illustrate what our public believes are potential major conflicts of interest for practicing surgeons and innovators.

Vignettes and Guidelines

The Professional Surgical Society Annual Meeting

While wandering the aisles of the "Adventures in New Surgery" meeting, a fetchingly attractive equipment representative asks if you want to have your golf swing analyzed "for free." You will also receive a memory stick with your golf swing video—if you only will spend some time in their booth. Your golf swing definitely has a nasty slice. Should you stop for some input? No, not unless you pay for the service.

There are reasons why these representatives are fetchingly attractive. The cost of swing analysis and a memory stick are trivial expenses to such a company. It is well worth the reward of capturing your attention, plus a pleasant interaction might prompt you to have reciprocal feelings of generosity toward them and their new product. Actually, it is well known in psychology and marketing circles that if you give a gift to someone, the receiver is quite inclined to return the favor. In fact, the return gift is usually more valuable than the first token [16, 17]. You are being baited and about to be hooked. It appears that the public and our lawmakers know that the science of marketing new products is far more refined than the average surgeon's awareness of these persuasive methods.

Here are some principles for surgeons to consider when feeling the conflict of marketing pressures:

1. How would this action (acceptance of gifts) look to your most critical grandmother? Not the nice grandma…the cranky, glass-half-full, paranoid, and persnickety one. This is your public.
2. Would you like to see your picture, with golf driver in hand and company logo in the background, on the front page of your local newspaper? The headline would read something like, "Rich Surgeon Takes Freebies From Billion Dollar Corporation."
3. Is the activity related to the surgical meeting? Can it be considered surgical education? (Isn't this why you have paid to attend?)
4. Is the gift of trivial value? You could hope that the actual cost to the company is less than $50, and thereby you might hope to sneak by with respect to AdvaMed guidelines. And after all, your golf swing needs help! But if you paid for this video analysis with the golf pro at The Club, it would cost you closer to $250.

Pay for it, or do not do it.

We will return to these four principles in the following vignettes: (1) Grandma's skeptical view, (2) Newspaper headlines, (3) Educational validity, and/or (4) Perceived value.

Detail Rep at your Office

The SurgiTool medical company representative stops by your office to see if she/he can bring lunch to your staff next week and to "see if there is anything your office needs. You'd be welcome to stop by for a quick bite, too." Should you give your approval? Your generous approval might allow you to repair bruised relationships with your office staff from last week's busy clinic. Plus, your office staff does not have the restrictive rules about potential conflicts of interest that you have. So, why not agree? You do not have to show up at all—the SurgiTool Rep has made that clear. No harm, no foul, right? Wrong. You are in charge of your clinic—or at least you hope to be seen as such. You own the actions of your clinic in the minds of others, including patients, even if you do not own the clinic on paper or in practice.

Do you remember the Privileges and Practice Agreement that you signed for your medical group and hospital? Do you remember that you belong to some very select and revered surgical societies? Both of these parties have strong views on industry-sponsored lunches and other freebies [13, 14]. Institutions are very specific about the accepted level of interaction between a device-maker representative and the physician using those devices. Moreover, your hospital, medical group, and professional societies know that (1) your grandma would think this is spurious; (2) the caption in the newspaper would be disparaging; (3) there is no real educational value to this event—it is just marketing; and (4) it will seem lavish to the rest of the world that does not enjoy free lunches.

New Equipment Rep in the Operating Room

The Mesh-It Corporation equipment representative meets you at the OR door and asks you to try out the company's new hernia mesh. "I noticed you had three hernia cases on today—all your colleagues love it," implicitly suggesting that you are behind current standards if you do not try it out for yourself. You are appropriately suspicious from the start, but also too generous with your time. Most ORs have a policy that if a surgeon really wants a special product, the OR will accommodate such a request for a trial period, but only if this request goes through proper channels. In some institutions, this approval process is seemingly endless—purposefully. Notably, the actual cost of the new mesh is rarely borne by the patient, hospital, surgeon, or anyone close to those who make purchasing decisions. (Is this a Medicare patient? Do you pay taxes?) The issues of pricing, costs, who pays, etc., are thankfully beyond the scope of this chapter.

What is your next step? It should be to say "No thanks." You would rather learn of new surgical advances through peer-reviewed journal articles and trusted surgical societies—like SAGES. You could ask for information to be left at the front desk. It might go right into the circular file (waste basket), but you will glance at it first…. maybe.

Let's review:

– Your granny will say, "Mesh is mesh, what's the big deal?"
– The headline will read something like, "Surgeons in Bed with Equipment Companies Drive Up Healthcare Costs."
– You would like to see a good, randomized trial presented at a SAGES meeting, with at least 10-year follow-up, but that is unlikely to happen. Remember what motivates for-profit companies? Profit.
– Whew! At least the product rep is not giving you money or food. That was easy.

Your Boss

It may be your hospital's CEO, CFO, CMO, or a Chairman named "Moe," who asks you to evaluate the new Zip-Zap closure device for the Officially Approved Devices Committee. In nearly the same breath, Moe mentions that the "NERL" building is very available for corporate naming sponsorship. (One can only hope that "NERL" is only a temporary acronym for the New and Expensive Research Labs.) Moe wonders aloud how nice it would be if the Zip-Zap company would want to donate enough for the naming rights to the NERL. Moe suggests, "Don't you already use Zip-Zap for your non-invasive [sic] procedures?" You can sense a gnawing tension inherent in this awkward juxtaposition of requests. Does the device approval process relate at all to the naming of research labs? "No!" says your good conscience…and federal law.

Not long ago, physicians and surgeons could own equity in their own pharmacies, supply houses, and/or treatment centers. The more one prescribed or ordered such drugs-devices-treatments, the more one profited— woo-hoo! (Remember Adam Smith's butcher? He was certain to prescribe an all-meat diet.) To the consternation of our funding lawmakers, American medical expenses have been rising year-over-year [18]. In simple logic (the fox guarding the henhouse), it has been legally decreed that providers and institutions should be separated from their inherent conflicts of interests [19]. This is why Medical Group bylaws are distinct and separate from Medical Center bylaws—though you may actually sit on committees for both.

Back to Moe's request: Should you evaluate the new product for your hospital's committee? It is hard to tell your chairperson "no," but you should be clear that accepting this duty has nothing to do with the very important challenge of funding and naming the research labs. "Good luck," you tell him, and "I'm glad it's your job to chase donors, not mine!"

To reframe the tenets of the Stark Regulations, aka the "Anti-Kickback Statute," in the principles above: (1) your grandma shoots foxes that come near her henhouse, (2) the newspaper will readily expose prescribing practices that might be seen as coupled to institutional fundraising, (3) you wish there would be some educational benefit to this effort, and (4) you are getting hungry just thinking about those endless late afternoon meetings. There better be good food!

Your Patient's Demands

A new patient comes to you with the specific request for a cholecystectomy using the new "scarless surgery" method that they have heard about. Maybe this patient is a professional model? You are a forward-thinking surgeon, who helps improve surgical practices—through appropriate registries, human clinical trials, and/or research projects. But you also know that surgery means scarring, even if it cannot be easily seen. How unfortunate it is that your hospital—separated by law from your ethical and financial concerns—put up that awkward billboard promoting "scarless surgery." Your hospital knows that if it is not continually marketing itself as "industry-leading," with all the newest devices, they will lose referrals and revenue. They might even portray Michelangelo himself as a surgeon if it would help sell their services.

The patient actually hands you a pamphlet about "Scarless Gallbladder Surgery" provided by your hospital. "This is what I want," she says. Getting back to your duties as her surgeon, you quickly learn that all the indications are there for her to undergo cholecystectomy, so you are ready to begin the operative consent process. Of course, you first want to clarify what your patient is expecting, versus what you are planning to recommend.

The operative consent process is critical. Unless you give your patient sufficient, unbiased information about your recommended treatment, its risks and benefits and alternatives—informed consent—you could be accused of not just malpractice, if something unexpected happens, but of an actual criminal act. It is called malpractice if you deviate from acceptable medical/surgical standards and that deviation causes harm, but it is criminal assault if you harm someone without an appropriate informed consent.

Need we say again:

– Your grandmother knows that surgery causes scars
– Newspapers love to sell papers—they will enlarge the color pictures
– Your patient will appreciate the unbiased education, as will an observing resident or student, and
– Your gallbladder is fine, so you are getting hungry.

Public Reporting by the Medical Device Industry

Did you know that medical device and pharmaceutical companies are required to keep track of the "freebies" that they give to physicians? The "Sunshine Act" can be seen as resulting from the loose oversight of our own past activities as physicians in this give-and-take arena [20]. While far from complete or precisely accurate, the online reporting may already list you on various company payrolls.

Currently, our surgical societies also collect such information, but usually without a dollar amount of "support" attached to each activity. The reporting is voluntary and unevenly scrutinized. These authors are unaware of any circumstance wherein conflict of interest self-reporting by surgical societies resulted in any substantial disciplinary action.

If these measures do not calm the ethical concerns of our public and lawmakers, the rigors of such data keeping and disclosure will only get more onerous. Your grandma knows what bribery looks like, and the newspapers will be quick to accuse companies and surgeons of collusion. The activities described in the vignettes above are marketing activities, not education. Do not skip your own breakfast.

CME Sessions vs. Non-CME, Industry Sponsored Events

Did you ever wonder why some industry "sponsored events" just across the hallway look very similar to the scientific presentations in the plenary room? They might even feature the same speaker, with very similar slides or videos. The same conclusion slide may be proposed in both presentations—that the ShaZam Tool is safe and effective.

But let's reflect a bit. You are not paying for the industry-sponsored event. Enticingly, they are serving robust refreshments, and you are hoping to quench your hunger for.... uh ... knowledge. But remember, equipment companies need robust product sales, not CME-accreditation. If these mirror-like "sponsored events" and exhibit hall booths were juxtaposed with the CME-granting scientific talks, it might get pretty darned confusing. That is why they are separated geographically, as required by ACCME guidelines. Should you go to the CME talk or attend the industry session and get some munchies? It is your choice, but note the badge scans or sign-in sheets. You are being tracked.

Your grandma will think you should skip the food and drink, since you could lose a few pounds anyway. The newspaper knows how to butter their bread—they have already sold advertising space to the very same company. Both talks may be educational, with their own perspectives, but the food won't really be that good.

Industry Courses for New Procedures

Do you have credentials and privileges to do "advanced laparoscopic procedures?" Now that you are out of residency and certifiably trained, don't you hope to stay current with new procedures and techniques? This process will often involve taking an industry-sponsored course, then getting "approved" by a variable process that assigns the delineation of privileges at each of your practice locations. Actually, some companies would prefer that you never be allowed to touch their expensive, investor-driven gadgets without first passing The Course—with food provided, of course. In fact, their captive session with you may actually be the *de facto* step required to acquire hospital privileges to use their equipment.

If you want to stay current, you will most likely be learning from those who have pioneered these new techniques or instrumentation. That is the way it has always been. Your job is to manage the inherent conflicts of interests in such relationships. To keep grandma, the newspapers, your bosses, and your surgical societies happy, you should check to be sure that:

1. The food and drink are sensible, not extravagant.
2. The event is held in appropriate surroundings, not a 5-star resort.

3. The instructors fully disclose their potential conflicts of interests.
4. You actually and verifiably learn what they purport to teach.

If the event does not have a pre- and post-test, and if no one is keeping track of the number of times you successfully complete the new procedure, you should be suspicious of the course's intent.

Trainee and Fellowship Funding

For many hospitals, training residents contribute to their operating budget (through Medicare part A subsidies). Consider this: If a resident earns $50,000/year and works 80 h/week, the pay is approximately $12/h—often for night and weekend work. That is great skilled labor at bargain prices for the hospital! But GME budgets do not supply enough resident salaries "to get all the work done." Whoops—they really meant to say, "to educate as many residents as we could."

Into this opportunity steps industry-sponsored research fellowships. For a medical device company, this represents effective R & D, plus very effective marketing to the trainee, all through one sponsored "educational salary." Fellowship positions in surgical training programs have grown, in concert with the zeal of introducing new devices into our surgical practices and becoming sub-specialists, while also partially filling the hospital staffing void brought on by restricted resident work hours. Fellowships are here to stay, and they need to be funded, and that creates some conflicts.

Your grandma wants more personalized attention and less talk of expensive gadgets during her pre-op visit. The newspapers have not caught up with this cause-and-effect training dilemma. One can only hope that surgical fellowships do not significantly dilute or delay the training of surgical residents. Residents and fellows would go hungry in order to do a good case.

Conclusions

Whether we are innovator-inventors, or mainstream users of well-marketed products, our public, our lawmakers, and our professional societies demand extra careful actions from every surgeon with respect to avoiding conflicts of interest. The authors suggest that our treasured patients deserve the full and unabashed disclosure of any potential conflict of interest that may affect our decisions and their decisions. They deserve unbiased, best practice care—the type that we would want provided to our most beloved relatives. Ethical surgical care requires full disclosure of real or perceived conflicts of interest, and to the extent possible, industry influence-free actions from all surgeons.

Disclosures

David Easter and Tazo Inui have no relevant conflicts of interest to report.

References

1. Davis L. J.B. Murphy: stormy petrel of surgery. New York: Van Rees Press; 1938. p. 155.
2. Ponsky JL. The development of PEG: how it was. J Interv Gastroenterol. 2011;1(2):88–9.
3. Chatterji AK, Fabrizio KR, Mitchell W, Schulman KA. Physician-industry cooperation in the medical device industry. Health Aff. 2008;27(6):1532–43.
4. Jamshidi R, et al. Magnamosis: magnetic compression anastomosis with comparison to suture and staple techniques. J Pediatr Surg. 2009;44(1):222–8.
5. Burton T. Do the FDA's regulations governing medical devices need to be overhauled? Wall Street J. 2015. http://www.wsj.com/articles/do-the-fdas-regulations-of-medical-devices-need-to-be-overhauled-1427079649?mod=ST1
6. Wee CC, et al. Quality of life among obese patients seeking weight loss surgery: the importance of obesity-related social stigma and functional status. J Gen Intern Med. 2013;28(2):231–8.
7. http://www.fda.gov/downloads/AdvisoryCommittees/CommitteesMeetingMaterials/MedicalDevices/MedicalDevicesAdvisoryCommittee/Gastroenterology-UrologyDevicesPanel/UCM302783.pdf
8. Nguyen NT, et al. Trends in use of bariatric surgery, 2003–2008. J Am Chem Soc. 2011;213(2):261–6.
9. AdvaMed Code of Ethics on Interactions with Health Care Professionals. http://advamed.org/res.download/112
10. Society for Vascular Surgery. Guidelines for interaction with industry. http://www.vascularweb.org/about/policies/Pages/guidelines-for-interaction-with-industry.aspx
11. American Association of Neurological Surgeons. https://www.aans.org/About%20AANS/~/media/D46157B93E9A481EB586F349392B6E8B.ashx
12. American Academy of Orthopedic Surgeons. Opinions on ethics and professionalism: the orthopedic surgeon's relationship with industry. http://www.aaos.org/about/papers/ethics/1204eth.asp

13. Strong VE, et al. Ethical considerations regarding the implementation of new technologies and techniques in surgery. Surg Endosc. 2014;28(8):2272–6.
14. Biffl WL, et al. Responsible development and application of surgical innovations: a position statement of the Society of University Surgeons. J Am Chem Soc. 2008;206(6):1204–9.
15. http://www.hhs.gov/healthcare/rights/law/
16. Fazal e Hasan S, Lings I, Neale L, Mortimer G. The role of customer gratitude in making relationship marketing investments successful. J Retail Consum Serv. 2014;21(5):788–96.
17. Cialdini RB. Influence: the psychology of persuasion. New York: Harper Business; 2006.
18. Peterson-Kaiser Health System Tracker. http://healthsystemtracker.org
19. Stark Law, 42 U.S.C. 1395nn. https://www.cms.gov/Medicare/Fraud-and-Abuse/PhysicianSelfReferral/index.html
20. http://cms.gov/openpayments

6. The FDA/CDRH Perspective on Device Innovation

Herbert Lerner and Martha W. Betz

- Strengthen the Clinical Trial Enterprise
    - Goal: Improve the efficiency, consistency, and predictability of the IDE process to reduce the time and number of cycles needed to reach appropriate IDE full approval for medical devices, in general, and for devices of public health importance, in particular.
    - Goal: Increase the number of early feasibility/first-in-human IDE studies submitted to FDA and conducted in the USA.
- Strike the Right Balance Between Premarket and Postmarket Data Collection
    - Goal: Assure the appropriate balance between premarket and postmarket data requirements to facilitate and expedite the development and review of medical devices, in particular high-risk devices of public health importance.
- Provide Excellent Customer Service

The three points noted above were presented to the staff of the Center for Devices and Radiological Health (CDRH) by Dr. Jeffrey Shuren, the Center Director, in early 2014 as the Center's 2014 Strategic Plan [1]. For those of us who work in CDRH and are tasked with the review of premarket applications for devices, the plan was an affirmation of many of the initiatives that had been implemented in the preceding few years at CDRH and which have been presented in the mission and vision of the Center: to protect and promote the public health and to assure that

© Springer International Publishing Switzerland 2016
S.C. Stain et al. (eds.), *The SAGES Manual Ethics
of Surgical Innovation*, DOI 10.1007/978-3-319-27663-2_6

patients in the USA have access to high-quality, safe, and effective medical devices of public health importance first in the world [2].

So how does all this happen? Surprisingly, many practicing physicians have no idea how the devices they use every day in their practices get to market or their responsibilities for reporting device malfunctions and adverse events.

FDA does not regulate the "practice of medicine." We do, however, have oversight of the drugs, biologics, tobacco products, and medical devices that are used for treating or diagnosing patients. The staff of CDRH is committed to working with industry to bring novel technologies to market and to meet the vision of the Center. In doing so, we encourage early and continuous communication with the review staff.

In the following sections, reference will be made to "Guidance" documents, which the FDA publishes to assist industry during device development and their interactions with the Agency. As sponsors develop new products, or clinicians begin a study with a new device or for a new indication, it is imperative that you read and understand these guidance documents. They provide the best current thinking that the agency has on a specific topic, and if followed, provide a predictable pathway to getting to market. You may note that some guidance documents are categorized as "draft" guidance, which are published to allow for public comment on a particular issue. Draft guidance documents are not intended for implementation purposes. Additionally, information is located on the FDA website in a section entitled "Device Advice" [3], which provides extensive information regarding device classification, content of submissions, and what to expect during the review process. Furthermore, the Division of Industry and Consumer Education (DICE) [4] is available as an educational resource to help those in the medical device industry and/or consumers understand FDA regulation and policies.

Getting New Devices to Market

Whether you are a young entrepreneur, an established innovator, or a practicing clinician who just had the "ah ha" moment in the OR for a new device to be used to treat patients, there is a regulatory pathway for getting the device to market. There are two main pathways for getting a device to market: premarket notification (510(k)) and premarket approval (PMA). In general, clinical data are necessary to demonstrate a reasonable assurance of safety and effectiveness for *de novo* and PMA applications; approximately 10 % of the 510(k)s we review require clinical data. Much of these clinical data are collected under an investigational device exemption (IDE), if conducted in the USA.

The discussions below will give the readers a better understanding of the regulatory process. As CDRH reviews the material submitted by sponsors, we remember the Center's priorities to bring safe and effective devices to market first in the world. In the following sections, we will briefly outline the regulatory pathways for sponsors to get their devices to market. Strategic planning is important so that each party, the sponsor and FDA, has all the information they need to maximize efficiency in the review process. The most important aspect to a successful relationship between the sponsor and FDA is open and frequent communication. Many clinical trials and application approvals have been delayed because of poor communication, and this can easily be avoided if there are open lines of communication and all discussions/decisions are written into the record.

To facilitate better communication between the involved parties, and based on experience from the pre-IDE process, the Agency published the guidance "Requests for Feedback on Medical Devices: The Pre-Submission Program and Meetings with FDA Staff" [5]. This guidance and program were developed to provide technical feedback on nonclinical or clinical testing methodologies used to support the different premarket submission areas. As described in the guidance, a presubmission is defined as "a written request for feedback from FDA to be provided in the form of a formal written response or, if the manufacturer chooses, a meeting or teleconference in which the feedback is documented in meeting minutes." FDA review staff have considered this program beneficial, especially when the packages have been well prepared by the sponsors and the questions are focused to ensure the efficiency of subsequent reviews, in particular the IDE review process. This has been especially helpful to sponsors as they proceed to the IRBs associated with their clinical sites.

The IDE

The IDE (Investigational Device Exemption) process [6] is generally the first formal step in getting new technologies studied in humans prior to marketing the device. Working with the FDA team of clinicians, scientists, and statisticians, sponsors develop the clinical trial design, statistical plan, study endpoints, and follow-up procedures for the data needed to support their marketing application. Depending on the nature of the technology and the risk to patients who might be exposed to the device, the trial may be of a short duration or much longer (e.g., months or years). The duration of the clinical study will impact when the marketing application should be submitted to FDA. Additionally, FDA may ask for stopping rules, interim analyses of the data, or other items to best protect the patients enrolled in the study. Once the data are collected, there are several paths to market, which will be outlined below. FDA also encourages sponsors to review our IDE guidance documents [7, 8] before submitting applications to the Agency. This will ensure better submissions and more efficiency in the review.

As noted above, one of the strategic goals for CDRH is to strengthen the Clinical Trial Enterprise and reduce the time and number of review cycles needed to reach appropriate full approval for IDEs. Within 9 months of implementing the program, September 2014, CDRH reduced the number of IDEs requiring more than two review cycles for approval by 34 % and reduced the overall median time by 53 % compared to 2013 [9]. Additionally, by mid-year 2015, CDRH aims to reduce the number of IDEs requiring more than two cycles to receive appropriate full approval decisions by 50 % in comparison with 2013 and reduce the overall median time to full appropriate approval to 30 days. The hope is to facilitate more timely investigation of devices, which should also result in increased access to devices of public health importance in a shorter time frame.

Premarket Notification

A premarket notification, also known as a 510(k), must be submitted to the FDA for a device that is not exempt from premarket review and for which a PMA is not required [10]. These devices are informally thought of as "me too" devices as they are compared to a previously cleared predicate device. The 510(k) submission should demonstrate that a device is at least as safe and effective as a legally marketed predicate device through comparison of the intended use and technological characteristics. Any differences and whether they alter the safety and effectiveness should be discussed and supported by any necessary performance data. A submission for a device determined to be substantially equivalent (SE) to the predicate can be legally marketed. Extensive information regarding the 510(k) process is located in the FDA guidance, "The 510(k) Program: Evaluating Substantial Equivalence in Premarket Notifications [510(k)]" [11].

The De Novo Classification Process

For devices that do not fall within an existing classification regulation or are not comparable to a device that is subject to the premarket approval process (described below), a *de novo* request may be appropriate if specific criteria are met. Briefly, a device should be low to moderate risk and be able to demonstrate a reasonable assurance of safety and effectiveness through the use of general and/or special controls as well as through risk mitigation [12]. Typical special controls may include specific performance testing, such as nonclinical or clinical testing, and labeling requirements. During the review process, the FDA will make a benefit-risk determination for the device [13]. Once the submission is reviewed, and the information is determined to be adequate to demonstrate a reasonable assurance of safety and effectiveness with the risks appropriately mitigated, the *de novo* can be granted and allow for marketing authorization. Granting a *de novo* request creates a new classification regulation, and the device can serve as a predicate for future devices to be reviewed through the 510(k) process.

In previous years, the law required a not substantially equivalent (NSE) determination due to a lack of predicate, new intended use, or different technological characteristics through the 510(k) process prior to submission of a *de novo*. However, the law was changed in July 2012 that allows a sponsor to submit a direct *de novo* classification request without having to have completed the 510(k) process. If a sponsor believes that this may be the appropriate pathway to market for their device, it is beneficial to submit a presubmission as described in the above section to facilitate early feedback from the FDA and determine whether the *de novo* process is appropriate for your device. There is also a significant amount of information publicly available on the CDRH Transparency website for *de novo* requests that have been granted marketing authorization that we would encourage a sponsor to preview prior to submission of a *de novo* request [14].

The PMA Process

A premarket approval (PMA) application is typically necessary for the highest class of medical devices, class III, where general and special controls are insufficient to reasonably assure safety and effectiveness. Class III medical devices are those that support or sustain human life, are of substantial importance in preventing impairment of human health, or present a potential, unreasonable risk of illness or injury [15]. The PMA submission should include summaries and in-depth reports of nonclinical and clinical testing as well as manufacturing information. A comprehensive list of PMA application contents is available on the FDA website as well as a number of device-specific guidance [16].

Once submitted, the PMA will be reviewed to ensure that valid scientific evidence has been provided to assure that the device is reasonably safe and effective for its intended use. If necessary, the FDA may refer the PMA to an outside panel of experts, known as an advisory committee, for review and hold a public meeting. If approved, the FDA may impose postapproval requirements, which may include continuing evaluation and periodic reporting on the safety, effectiveness, and reliability of the device. As noted above for other marketing submissions, it is beneficial to submit a presubmission to elicit early feedback from CDRH on your PMA submission package to facilitate the review process.

Humanitarian Device Exemption

A less frequently used pathway to market a device is the Humanitarian Device Exemption (HDE). An HDE may be submitted for humanitarian use devices that are intended to benefit patients by treating or diagnosing a disease or condition in fewer than 4,000 individuals in the United States per year. An HDE application is similar to a PMA application, but the data are not required to meet the same effectiveness requirements. Instead, an HDE should demonstrate that the device does not pose an unreasonable risk or illness or injury, and that the probable benefit to health outweighs the risk of injury or illness from its use, when considering probable risks and benefits of currently available devices or alternative forms of treatment [17].

FDA/CDRH and Innovation

In 2011, the FDA implemented the Entrepreneurs-in-Residence Program to assist the Agency with "big picture" issues affecting the medical device industry. The goal of this program was to include members from industry, academia, venture capital, and research to assist FDA staff to streamline a regulatory pathway for innovative devices [18]. This program helped initiate the Innovation Pathway described below and also looked to streamline clinical trials, striking the right balance between pre- and postmarket data requirements for devices. Furthermore, the FDA has started the Network of Experts, which is a vetted group of outside scientists, clinicians, and engineers who provide supplemental expertise to FDA staff on new and emerging fields of science and pioneering technologies [19]. Through these programs, as well as implementation of the Early Feasibility Medical Device enterprise, CDRH has made progress to increase availability of novel medical devices in the USA.

Specifically, the FDA issued an Early Feasibility Guidance [20] in October 2013 to stimulate the initiation of "first-in-human" studies being performed in the USA to attempt to get novel devices utilized and intended to help bring new devices to US patients earlier. As noted above, the first goal of the Center's strategic plan is to strengthen the Clinical Trial enterprise, and to help achieve that goal, the Center created novel approaches for industry to bring their devices for review including the early feasibility program. FDA recognizes that clinical testing has gone "offshore" due to costs associated with doing clinical studies in the USA, as well as the time needed to get an IDE through the FDA review process. This created a lag in the availability of beneficial medical devices for US patients, as well as the costs of not having these technologies available to those who might have benefited from such technologies.

As outlined in the guidance, an early feasibility IDE may be appropriate when nonclinical testing methods are not available or adequate to provide necessary information for device development and clinical data are required. Specifically, earlier clinical use of the device in a limited number of subjects is needed to provide better insight into the clinical safety and device function, revise subsequent clinical and nonclinical testing, and improve device performance through iteration before finalizing the design. Additionally, approval of an early feasibility IDE study may be based on less nonclinical data, as exhaustive testing would not likely provide necessary information for device development, although additional patient protection measures may be necessary.

Continuous dialogue between the sponsor and FDA will allow a review of the data from the first smaller cohort of patients, allows the sponsor to make iterative changes to the device, and allows both parties to assess the initial risks associated with the device and make changes to the investigational plan. Another important component of the Early Feasibility process is that the sponsor can complete some of the nonclinical testing, which had been deferred to allow final device design, and for which the data can be assessed after the initiation of the clinical trial.

Using this approach, FDA and the sponsor can hopefully bring new devices to market earlier. The Early Feasibility Guidance includes new approaches to facilitate timely device and clinical protocol modification during the early feasibility study. After the completion of the early feasibility study, the sponsor can then choose to expand the study to a traditional feasibility study to assess the device in a larger number of patients or they can submit a formal pivotal study, assuming that the data support the clinical use of the device and the appropriate nonclinical data to embark upon a pivotal study with greater patient exposure have been completed.

Additionally, in 2011 FDA initiated the *Innovation Pathway* to facilitate the development and expedite the review of breakthrough technologies that address unmet public health needs [21]. The goal of this program was to engage with innovators much earlier and more interactively during device development in the hope of reducing the time and cost of bringing new, safe, and effective technologies to patients. In 2012, sponsors of novel technologies were encouraged to apply to the Innovation Pathway program, and several device groups with novel technologies in end-stage renal disease were selected to participate. Working together, these technologies were reviewed and device development plans and clinical trials were initiated. From the lessons learned with this limited endeavor, FDA has developed new draft guidance [22] for devices intended for life-threatening or irreversibly debilitating diseases, which is intended to incorporate some of the principles piloted as part of the Innovation Pathway.

Expedited Access for Premarket Approval Medical Devices Intended for Unmet Medical Need

CDRH recently published a draft guidance, "Expedited Access for Premarket Approval Medical Devices Intended for Unmet Medical Need for Life Threatening or Irreversibly Debilitating Diseases or Conditions" [22]. Although this guidance is not for implementation currently, it represents CDRH's current thinking. In this draft guidance, CDRH has proposed a pathway for novel technologies to reach patients in a timelier manner while continuing to meet the statutory standard for PMA approval.

To be eligible for the Expedited Access Program (EAP), there are three criteria which must be met:

1. The device is intended to treat or diagnose a life-threatening or irreversibly debilitating disease of condition
2. The device must meet at least one of the following criteria:

   (a) No approved alternative treatment or means of diagnosis exists.
   (b) The device represents a breakthrough technology that provides a clinically meaningful advantage over existing approved technology available on the market.
   (c) The device offers significant, clinically meaningful advantages over existing approved alternatives.

3. The sponsor submits an acceptable draft Data Development Plan.

How will this be accomplished? One aspect of the EAP is to facilitate appropriate engagement of management as well as shifting from the normal practice of device application review to allow FDA to consider shifting the balance of data required for these technologies from the premarket to the postmarket [23], as well as accepting a greater degree of uncertainty in the benefit-risk profile as outlined in the Agency's "Factors to Consider When Making Benefit-Risk Determinations in Medical Device Pre-Market Approvals and De Novo Classifications" Guidance document. In each application, FDA and the sponsor will review the new technology, assess the potential risks, identify the mitigations for those risks, and develop the appropriate regulatory pathway for the device.

The Federal Food, Drug, and Cosmetic Act (the Act) does specifically state that "In making a determination of a reasonable assurance of the *effectiveness* of a device...the secretary shall consider whether the extent of data that otherwise would be required for approval of the application with respect to effectiveness can be reduced through reliance on postmarket controls." This also aligns with the "least burdensome" provisions of the Act and correlates strongly with the Center's strategic priorities related to ensuring the right balance between pre- and postmarket data collection to facilitate and expedite the development and review of medical devices, in particular high-risk devices of public health importance.

SAGES and FDA

As discussed previously, FDA does not regulate the practice of medicine; we are, however, interested in the new techniques of surgical intervention (i.e., NOTES, POEM) associated with the use of already marketed devices.

To facilitate the interaction of industry, investigators and FDA, there are several pathways to consider. In general, these will allow FDA to work with all involved to design a robust clinical (IDE) trial or to assure that the data are sufficient to expand an indication for an already marketed device.

- SAGES Emerging Technology session at the annual meeting provides a platform for new innovation to be presented and discussed. FDA would be interested in participating at this session.
- SAGES Technology and Value Assessment Committee may also be a place for early discussion of new technologies, perhaps in response to unusual clinical outcomes with marketed devices or off-label use of a device. FDA is already represented on the committee and would be happy to expand its role.
- FDA understands that there are situations when we must go outside the Agency to find expertise for some of our clinical trial initiatives or for guidance during our advisory panels. SAGES participates in our Network of Experts; however, to help FDA with ensuring that we have appropriate clinical expertise available, we encourage SAGES members to become Special Government Employees (SGEs). SGEs can assist the FDA during advisory panel meetings when we are seeking additional perspectives on device-specific matters, as well as provide critical thinking on difficult issues not related to a particular device submission.
- Invite FDA to your meetings, either the annual meeting or specific workshops, etc., so that we have an understanding of major issues, some of which may eventually come to us for review.
- Medical Device (MDR) Reporting. The best way for FDA to assess signals for device issues is through the use of our MDR reporting system. This is a voluntary, online system where any malfunction, adverse event, or other device-related issue can be reported to FDA. Our signal management team can look for trends associated with a device, and we can then take appropriate

action, working with the manufacturer, to alleviate the issue. This is a critical tool that the FDA utilizes and we encourage your colleagues and hospitals/clinics to become familiar with MDR reporting.

• Finally, as noted in the Strategic Plan for CDRH, customer service is important to us. Feel free to pick up the phone or e-mail someone at FDA if you have questions about our procedures, and use the guidance documents outlined above as a good reference to help you get started. We encourage you to work through SAGES committees to identify global issues and include FDA participation in future discussions.

References

1. 2014–2015 Strategic Priorities. http://www.fda.gov/downloads/AboutFDA/Centers Offices/OfficeofMedicalProductsandTobacco/CDRH/CDRHVisionandMission/UCM431016.pdf

2. CDRH Mission, Vision and Shared Values. http://www.fda.gov/AboutFDA/Centers Offices/OfficeofMedicalProductsandTobacco/CDRH/ucm300639.htm. June 2014.

3. Device Advice: Comprehensive Regulatory Assistance. http://www.fda.gov/MedicalDevices/DeviceRegulationandGuidance/. October 2014.

4. Contact Us – Division of Industry and Consumer Education. http://www.fda.gov/MedicalDevices/DeviceRegulationandGuidance/ContactUs--DivisionofIndustryandConsumerEducation/ucm20041265.htm. January 2015.

5. Requests for Feedback on Medical Device Submissions: The Pre-Submission Program and Meetings with Food and Drug Administration Staff. http://www.fda.gov/downloads/medicaldevices/deviceregulationandguidance/guidancedocuments/ucm311176.pdf. February 2014.

6. Device Advice: Investigational Device Exemption (IDE). http://www.fda.gov/MedicalDevices/DeviceRegulationandGuidance/HowtoMarketYourDevice/InvestigationalDeviceExemptionIDE/. June 2014.

7. FDA Decisions for Investigational Device Exemption Clinical Investigations. http://www.fda.gov/downloads/MedicalDevices/DeviceRegulationandGuidance/GuidanceDocuments/UCM279107.pdf. August 2014.

8. IDE Guidance. http://www.fda.gov/MedicalDevices/DeviceRegulationandGuidance/HowtoMarketYourDevice/InvestigationalDeviceExemptionIDE/ucm162453.htm. June 2014.

9. Faris, Owen. Strengthening the medical device clinical trial enterprise. http://www.fda.gov/downloads/Training/CDRHLearn/UCM431045.pdf

10. Premarket Notification (510k). http://www.fda.gov/MedicalDevices/DeviceRegulationandGuidance/HowtoMarketYourDevice/PremarketSubmissions/PremarketNotification510k/default.htm. August 2014.

11. The 510(k) Program: Evaluation Substantial Equivalence in Premarket Notifications [510(k)]. http://www.fda.gov/downloads/MedicalDevices/.../UCM284443.pdf. July 2014.

12. *De Novo* Classification Process (Evaluation of Automatic Class III Designation) Draft Guidance. http://www.fda.gov/downloads/MedicalDevices/DeviceRegulationand Guidance/GuidanceDocuments/UCM273903.pdf. DRAFT Guidance (not currently for implementation), August 2014.

13. Factors to Consider When Making Benefit-Risk Determinations in Medical Device Premarket Approval and *De Novo* Classifications. http://www.fda.gov/downloads/ MedicalDevices/DeviceRegulationandGuidance/GuidanceDocuments/UCM296379. pdf. March 2012.

14. Evaluation of Automatic Class III Designation (De Novo) Summaries. http://www. fda.gov/AboutFDA/CentersOffices/OfficeofMedicalProductsandTobacco/CDRH/ CDRHTransparency/ucm232269.htm. February 2015.

15. Premarket Approval (PMA). http://www.fda.gov/Medicaldevices/Deviceregulation andguidance/Howtomarketyourdevice/Premarketsubmissions/remarketapprovalpma/ Default.Htm. August 2014.

16. PMA Guidance Documents. http://www.fda.gov/MedicalDevices/DeviceRegulation andGuidance/HowtoMarketYourDevice/PremarketSubmissions/Premarket ApprovalPMA/ucm143067.htm. September 2013.

17. Humanitarian Device Exemption. http://www.fda.gov/MedicalDevices/ DeviceRegulationandGuidance/HowtoMarketYourDevice/PremarketSubmissions/ HumanitarianDeviceExemption/. DRAFT Guidance (not currently for implementation) June 2014.

18. Entrepreneurs in Residence Program. http://www.fda.gov/AboutFDA/CentersOffices/ OfficeofMedicalProductsandTobacco/CDRH/CDRHInnovation/InnovationPathway/ ucm286138.htm. June 2014.

19. CDRH Network of Experts. http://www.fda.gov/AboutFDA/CentersOffices/ OfficeofMedicalProductsandTobacco/CDRH/ucm289534.htm. October 2014.

20. Investigational Device Exemptions (IDEs) for Early Feasibility Medical Device Clinical Studies, Including Certain First in Human (FIH) Studies. http://www.fda.gov/ downloads/medicaldevices/deviceregulationandguidance/guidancedocuments/ ucm279103.pdf. October 2013.

21. Innovation Pathway. http://www.fda.gov/AboutFDA/CentersOffices/Officeof MedicalProductsandTobacco/CDRH/CDRHInnovation/InnovationPathway/default. htm. March 2014.

22. Expedited Access for Premarket Approval Medical Devices Intended for Unmet Medical Need for Life Threatening or Irreversibly Debilitating Diseases or Conditions Draft Guidance. http://www.fda.gov/downloads/MedicalDevices/DeviceRegulation andGuidance/GuidanceDocuments/UCM393978.pdf. DRAFT Guidance (not currently for implementation), April 2014.

23. Balancing Premarket and Postmarket Data Collection for Devices Subject to Premarket Approval. http://www.fda.gov/downloads/MedicalDevices/Device RegulationandGuidance/GuidanceDocuments/UCM393994.pdf. DRAFT Guidance (not currently for implementation), April 2014.

7. The FDA and Surgical Innovation

S.D. Schwaitzberg and C.J. Schwaitzberg

The United States is the largest single medical device market in the world representing more than a third of the global market which might reach as much as $133 billion by 2016. Most of the 6500 medical device companies in the USA are small- or medium-sized businesses with less than 50 employees [1]. A significant percentage of these small businesses are startups with a little or no revenue. These small businesses are the lifeblood of innovation that has been responsible for the preeminent position that the USA has enjoyed thus far. The characteristics of the innovation pathway are critical to the success of device development, improvements in health, and cost-effectiveness of care in this country. Although the FDA stands as the first significant gatekeeper in the innovation process, this innovation pathway has several components in addition, such as the impact of CPT coding, payers, group pricing, training, and the like. Medical devices are reviewed in the Center for Devices and Radiological Health (CDRH), which was established under another name in 1976 after the US Congress passed the Medical Device Amendments to the Federal Food, Drug, and Cosmetic Act. Today, the FDA employs more than 14,000 full-time equivalents (FTE), of which approximately 1400 work in the CDRH [2].

© Springer International Publishing Switzerland 2016
S.C. Stain et al. (eds.), *The SAGES Manual Ethics of Surgical Innovation*, DOI 10.1007/978-3-319-27663-2_7

The Role of CDRH

According their website "the mission of the Center for Devices and Radiological Health (CDRH) [of the FDA] is to protect and promote the public health. We assure that patients and providers have timely and continued access to safe, effective, and high-quality medical devices and safe radiation-emitting products. We provide consumers, patients, their caregivers, and providers with understandable and accessible science-based information about the products we oversee. We facilitate medical device innovation by advancing regulatory science, providing industry with predictable, consistent, transparent, and efficient regulatory pathways, and assuring consumer confidence in devices marketed in the U.S" [3]. Careful reading of this mission can give insight into the balance of issues which, at times, seem to be at cross purposes. For instance, the word "timely" is balanced against the need to make determinations of whether a device is safe, effective, and high quality. To this end, how much time for this process is reasonable? This question has been debated in numerous forums. On the one hand, the concept that *time is money* creates a downward pressure on the device industry. This pressure drives applicants to the FDA processes to get through this set of procedures as quickly as possible and move on to the other challenges to the innovation pathway – such as the acquisition of a level I CPT code (if needed) or approval by the payers. This perceived excessive tightness of the sieve by the medical device industry is balanced against charges by patient advocacy groups that the federal system is too lax and that patients are placed at risk as a result. FDA officials clearly find themselves in the middle of a conundrum which can be further complicated by potential political pressure that ensues when a high profile device is found to perform more poorly than predicted.

Device Approval: Process Problems and Opportunities

In the surgical/endoscopic arena, there are two basic ways we can consider how devices move through the regulatory pathway. Within these basic considerations, there are multiple subsets which add further complexity outside the scope of this writing. One way to consider an individual device is to consider whether the individual device represents a tool or procedure. This distinction is important because of the levels of evidence needed to secure FDA approval or clearance for marketing. As a general rule, when an investigational device represents a new procedure this constitutes a Class III device and the level of evidence needed for introduction to the marketplace is substantial. The premarket approval process (PMA) requires substantial clinical evidence through the clinical trial process. In fact, to use these devices on human subjects the device must be granted an investigational device exemption (IDE) in order to secure approval by investigational review boards (IRB) and initiate the clinical trial. When the new medical device is a tool used to facilitate standard of care clinical procedures the burden of proof has more to do with the operational performance of the device itself relative to the claims made by the manufacturer.

A second way to consider these devices is based on originality of the device (not to be confused with patentability). The 510(k) process allows manufacturers to submit a pre-market notification on Class II or lower devices, requesting the FDA clear products for marketing based on the argument that the proposed device is *substantially equivalent* to a previous device generally referred to as the "predicate device". This process can be fairly rapid but can also be subject to significant controversy since the definition of substantial equivalence can be open to interpretation. Furthermore, the substantial equivalence process can be iterated, leaving one to wonder at times whether or not the recently approved device is really substantially equivalent to the original predicate device approved several generations of the 510(k) process previously. The 510(k) process can be applied to either tools or procedural devices.

In part the criticisms of the 510(k) process stem from the facts that the finding of substantial equivalence does not mean a priori that clinical effective and safety can be surmised in the absence of clinical data on the device in question. Furthermore, in combination with an iteration paradigm, the opportunity for errors in judgment is magnified. For instance, the performance of a device in location A may not accurately predict the performance of a similar device in location B. This combination of events is demonstrated in the recent recall of certain transvaginal tape (TVT) products placed for urinary incontinence. The predicate device was approved based on substantial equivalence of the sling fabric safety record in cardiac surgery. Additional preclinical evidence based on rat studies was submitted with the application in order to garner approval for this urologic indication. Within 2 years, a second transvaginal tape product was approved, with the first product cited as the predicate device. An unfortunate series of events ensued, resulting in the withdrawal from the market of the first device – but not resulting in any consideration of action to potentially remove secondary devices based on the original approval from the market. A significant number of complications have developed in patients who received the subsequent devices as well, with more than 12,000 claims filed against various manufacturers for complications of pain and mesh erosion [4, 5]. The extreme example of this process is revealed in the history of the De Puy ASR XL acetabular component, which was approved by the FDA in 2008. Ardaugh et al. chronicled the ancestry of this device in the *New England Journal of Medicine* across a 50-year history through 95 devices and varying iterations of femoral heads and acetabular components, many of which do not resemble the final product. The original predicate products that were developed prior to 1976 had been removed from the market long before the 2008 approval because of poor clinical effectiveness and high risk of revision [6].

Since these mesh products were previously classified as Class II products, the current regulations do not require a PMA (premarket approval) along with a clinical trial to assess safety and effectiveness independently of potential predicate devices. There has been subsequent discussion to move these devices to Class III where more stringent controls apply.

Clearly, these are examples from the far end of the spectrum of the 510(k) process and represent only a fraction of thousands of approved products, most of which perform as expected. The high-profile nature of these examples impacting more than 100,000 people has certainly ignited prominent organizations to question process as a whole. Many of these impacted patients required revisional surgery(s), device explant, and significant pain management. In 2011, the Institute of Medicine issued a report: *Medical Devices and the Public's Health: The FDA 510(k) Clearance Process at 35 Years* – The committee opined that the 510(k) process was created on a flawed regulatory framework and should be rebuilt as an integrated premarket and postmarket regulatory system based on somewhat general principles of evidence, transparency, predictability, innovation, and public safety. No specific recommendations were made at that time [7].

The FDA CDRH responded with seven suggestions aimed at improving the scope, authority, and accountability of the process to include greater post-market surveillance and the opportunity to rescind previous 510(k) clearance when appropriate.

There is no doubt that members within CDRH recognize many of the flaws of the system. However, they function under a regulatory framework which in the federal bureaucracy is basis for determinations and decision-making. Clearly, the discussion has spawned interest in revising the regulatory framework in order to evolve into a more optimal system.

Should the FDA Regulate Surgery?

The FDA/CDRH is not charged with the direct regulation of specific surgical procedures at this time. However, indirect regulation does in fact occur through the labeling, which specifies the intended use of certain products and devices. The conduct of a Nissen fundoplication for reflux is not governed by the FDA. This is true regardless of whether the procedure is performed laparoscopically or via an incision. All of the tools used in these procedures are approved for *general use* within the abdomen and could be used to remove a kidney as well. On the other hand, the slurry of endolumenal devices developed specifically for use in the treatment of reflux are considered Class III devices, and regulations require the FDA to review clinical trial data prior to approval. If approvable, the language around the devices' labeling becomes a critical issue since the scope of use becomes defined and subsequent changes may require further clinical data. An example of this was seen recently when the manufacturer of one of the laparoscopic banding devices wished to expand the indications to a lower body mass index group than specified in the original approval. The approval for expansion of the indications was based on a very defined set of questions to which the clinical trial was addressed regardless of what other data might be available. These scenarios can create some dissonance between what is approvable by the FDA and what payers (government or private) might or might not choose to reimburse surgeons based on these new indications. The battleground can become quite muddy when there is temptation to limit the clinical indications of what might be considered a tool to a specific clinical procedure. This is exemplified in the case of the surgical robot which was approved initially as a tool for general use, similar to laparoscopy, based on the fact that the tasks were broken down to common denominators such as grasping, cutting, traction, and the like. Thus it is remarkable that when the robotic approach was combined with single incision laparoscopy (both approved for general use) that the approval labeling extended no further than single-port robotic cholecystectomy. On the surface, it is a completely reasonable procedure in terms of safety and effectiveness, but it is arguably not an ideal procedure to perform robotically in terms of overall value yet. The critical issue here is whether or not it is desirable to have the FDA approve tools on a procedure-by-procedure basis. The concept that new determinations concerning the levels of evidence for approval on a per-procedural basis would need to be developed and applied would certainly be concerning to medical device companies, as the cost of performing these multiple trial could be prohibitive. This would allow the FDA fairly broad oversight on the practice of surgery if applied in the strictest sense. The FDA is not mandated to regulate the practice of medicine. Some would argue that the level of safety would increase based on high-profile reports of injury that reach the public eye; however, many critics are unable to discern whether these are device failures or surgeon performance failures. On the other hand, criticism that medical device innovation is currently being stifled in the USA by an over-burdensome regulatory process (to be fair, the reimbursement process must be included in this criticism) could be valid as well. Both sides of the issue are important: patient safety is clearly paramount but at the same time, the idea that we can innovate without any risk is simply untrue. We must seek new ways to mitigate risk associated with medical device innovation. Recent interest by the FDA simulation training for some of these potentially riskier new devices that go through the PMA (but not 510(k) process is aimed at this problem and is manifested by approval for some endovascular devices be accompanied by the development of an appropriate simulation training prior to clinical use by individuals. This has been operationalized in certain endolumenal vascular catheterization devices, raising certain future questions about the need to garner FDA approval for simulation devices, particularly if they are tied to specific instruments. The level of evidence needed to validate a simulator in terms of transfer of training would be complicated for new devices and might potentially delay market introduction of the actual device. There is no mechanism to insert these requirements into clearance requirements for devices reviewed through the 501(k) mechanism.

The Role of the FDA in the Innovation Pathway

Certainly, if it is the mission of the FDA CDRH center to facilitate timely device innovation, an analysis of the predictability and transparency of the regulatory pathways (in the context of patient safety) compared to those processes used in other parts of the world can be performed. The European Union, for example, apparently has a substantially different take on medical device regulation, which some laud for leading to faster approval for new devices and others criticize for being too lax. The EU has no single unified oversight body responsible for regulation of medical and surgical devices. Instead, it maintains several Directives on standards for devices and mandates that its member states each appoint competent (governmental or private/for-profit) certification authorities, referred to as "notified bodies", to oversee and confirm that EU standards are being met. These directives outline four classes of device: Class I devices are those that are considered low-risk, such as sticking plasters or corrective glasses. This class of device can, with a few exceptions, be marketed solely with self-certification by the device manufacturer. Class IIa devices are medium-low risk devices, such as tracheal tubes, which require oversight by the notified body during the production stage. Class IIb and III devices are medium- and high-risk devices, respectively, and require inspection at both the design and manufacturing stages [8]. Class III devices also require "explicit prior authorization with regard to conformity" to be placed on the market [9].

Once approved by any notified body in any EU member state, a device is considered approved for circulation in all EU member states. This style of regulation is known in the EU as a "New Approach" directive. Several other products in the EU, such as pressure vessels and personal protective equipment, are also regulated through New Approach standards [10]. This allows each EU member state to regulate its devices semi-autonomously and without a cumbersome EU bureaucracy, while still maintaining a level of connection to other member states in the Union.

Due to these and several other differences between the FDA and EU processes for device regulation, the European system is often quicker to approve higher-risk devices than the FDA, getting patients access to these innovations more quickly. This may be due to the fact that the FDA requires evidence of both safety and efficacy of a device, whereas a European CE Mark only requires proof that a device is safe and that it performs in a manner consistent with the manufacturer's intended use [11]. However, this very efficiency of approval that has come under fire from the FDA, who in an unreleased internal 2012 report condemningly entitled "Unsafe and Ineffective Devices Approved in the EU that were Not Approved in the US". Following a highly publicized mishap in which 80,000 European women received breast implants made with industrial-grade silicone rather than the required medical-grade material, the FDA criticized the EU's use of private regulatory bodies and low requirements for patient safety and efficacy studies [12]. Clearly, the contrast between the European and American systems shows the consequences that differing opinions on the relative merits of Safety and Efficiency can have for patients and for the medical device industry.

When a device is subject to approval by the PMA process, an advisory panel may be constituted to assist the FDA in non-binding fashion in making final determinations concerning approval and labeling. The panels consist of expert clinicians as well as representative from the community and industry. The panels are a matter of public record and are charged with the responsibilities of reviewing all of the data submitted to the FDA and of participating in the hearing process. There has been controversy concerning which experts should sit on these panels: a 2007 federal ruling added limitations to the participation of any panel member who has any financial interest of a device under consideration. The financial conflict of interest issues are obvious, yet critics of this policy – including three United States Senators (from states with significant medical device manufacturing activity) – cite of the lack of expertise on these panels as contributing to the increasing bottleneck of innovation in the United States since the policy was initiated [13]. Many votes are straightforward, yet others are far more complex as members find themselves pondering the questions of "How much risk can be tolerated for a given level of benefit?" before voting. Often, decisions are made in a vacuum where panelists make educated guesses at these issues based on their expertise. In the last few years, these issues are highlighted by the new (endolumenal) devices proposed for the treatment of morbid obesity. Each of these devices will be associated with a unique profile of reduction of excess weight as well a unique risk profile. The dilemma for a panelist contemplating approval is centered around questions like "What does the public want?" and "What is the public risk tolerance?". Lerner et al. at the FDA surveyed patient to assess this question in weight loss devices. This provides a tool for payers, FDA panelists, and the medical device industry to understand what risk/benefit space a device might fit into relative to what a relevant population is looking for. As expected, effectiveness and risk tolerance do travel together where less effective devices should present risk profiles similar to medical management. However, in a follow-up editorial Talamini pointed out how significant and surprising this type of data might be: "…devices aiming for significant excess weight loss similar to currently approved devices such as the Realize gastric band, the Lap-Band carry a higher potential benefit and therefore would be permitted a greater degree of risk. Patients appear willing to assume that risk. An FDA survey demonstrated that obese patients would be willing to tolerate a *fivefold risk of death* to increase weight loss from 5 to 20 %." [14, 15].

The FDA should be applauded for this creative approach since the value of these data is obvious. This paradigm needs to be replicated across more domains which may represent opportunity for the major societies to partner with the FDA. As new medical and surgical innovations reach the markets these studies must be repeated since disruptive innovation may impact the risk tolerance of the target population. Another valuable innovation is the FDA MAUDE database (https://www.accessdata.fda.gov/scripts/cdrh/cfdocs/cfmaude/search.cfm), which serves as a repository of device information relating to failures and complications. This is accessible to the public via the Internet. Reporting is voluntary and clearly underrepresents potential problems, but is a step in the right direction as it may serve as an early warning notification when used by surgeons.

These concepts lead us to a more nuanced appreciation of the dilemma. It is not a simple question of whether the approval process is too fast to be safe or too slow, crippling the device industry in the context of making sure no patient comes to harm (Fig. 7.1). Just as discussions are moving towards population rather than individual outcomes, federal agencies have a duty to the public as a whole. A device mired in

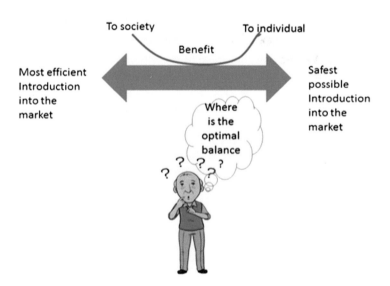

Fig. 7.1. The safest possible introduction for the individual may not represent the greatest societal benefit. Achieving equipoise so that there is safe market introduction via a process that is not overly burdensome is a challenging task.

an endless regulatory process might result in an application withdrawal or a bankrupt company. This is not necessarily of great concern unless this device would have relieved pain, reduced cost, or lessened morbidity if introduced in a timely fashion. What of the jobs lost or never created? At the same, a utilitarian "needs of the many" approach could be fraught with unacceptable individual abuse. Complete risk elimination is unachievable in the portfolio of interventional devices, but effective risk mitigation should be possible. This is really not different than a clinical scenario where the factors of patient selection and procedure appropriateness are balanced against the known risks. The patient cannot mandate a complication-free experience but does have a reasonable expectation that their procedure will be conducted with great expertise and care. Similarly, the device industry deserves an efficient process. This does not mean the fastest approval least expensive since rapid but poorly done work may not be the most cost effective or associated with subsequent and costly risk mitigation.

Conclusion

Surgeons should appreciate that the general mandate of the FDA is a critical component of innovation and safe device use. Most surgeons depend on FDA analysis of safety and effectiveness since they are incapable and generally unwilling to do these analyses for themselves. There are clear opportunities for improvement and there is evidence of continuous movement towards this. The federal government must be certain to provide adequate staffing both in numbers and talent. Recent increases in user fees are aimed at accomplishing this. As surgeons or lay citizens, we should be willing to volunteer our time and expertise to participate in the advisory process. Finally, there is abundant evidence that valuable information on medical devices resides in silos which, when brought to light of day, will assist both physicians and the public in their approaches to balancing the risks of medical devices and interventional procedures.

References

1. The Medical Device Industry in the United States. http://selectusa.commerce.gov/industry-snapshots/medical-device-industry-united-states. Accessed 2 May 2015.
2. Food and Drug Administration Distribution of Full-Time Equivalent (FTE) Employment Program Level. http://www.fda.gov/downloads/AboutFDA/ReportsManualsForms/Reports/BudgetReports/UCM301553.pdf. Accessed 17 May 2015.

3. Mission and Vision of the FDA. http://www.fda.gov/downloads/AboutFDA/Centers Offices/OfficeofMedicalProductsandTobacco/CDRH/CDRHVisionandMission/ UCM384576.pdf. Accessed 12 May 2015,

4. Cohen R, Orr JS. A surefire profit-maker could cost its maker dearly. http://www. nj.com/specialprojects/index.ssf?/specialprojects/implants/implantsside2.html. Accessed 1 June 2015.

5. 510(k); Pathway for Safer drugs or Recipe for Disaster. http://brandilawblog. com/2013/06/03/510k-pathway-for-safer-drugs-or-recipe-for-disaster/. Accessed 10 May 2015.

6. Ardaugh BM, Graves SE. Redberg the 510(k) ancestry of a metal-on-metal hip implant. N Engl J Med. 2013;368:97–100.

7. Institute of Medicine. Medical devices and the public's health: the FDA 510(k) clearance process at 35 years – http://iom.nationalacademies.org/Reports/2011/Medical-Devices-and-the-Publics-Health-The-FDA-510k-Clearance-Process-at-35-Years/ Report-Brief.aspx#sthash.yY6mU9lW.dpufhttp://iom.nationalacademies.org/ Reports/2011/Medical-Devices-and-the-Publics-Health-The-FDA-510k-Clearance-Process-at-35-Years/Report-Brief.aspx-sthash.yY6mU9lW.dpuf

8. European Commission. Regulation of the European Parliament and of the Council on medical devices, and amending Directive 2001/83/EC, Regulation (EC) No 178/2002 and Regulation (EC) No 1223/2009. http://ec.europa.eu/health/medical-devices/files/ revision_docs/proposal_2012_542_en.pdf. Accessed 19 July 2015.

9. The Council of the European communities. Council Directive 93/42/EEC of 14 June 1993 concerning medical devices. http://eur-lex.europa.eu/legal-content/EN/ TXT/?uri=CELEX:31993L0042. Accessed 19 July 2015.

10. Sorrel S. Medical Device Development: U.S. and EU Differences Less stringent requirements in the European Union result in faster medical device approval times. http://www.appliedclinicaltrialsonline.com/medical-device-development-us-and-eu-differences. Accessed 19 July 2015.

11. Chi C. Which way to go: CE mark or FDA approval? http://www.mdtmag.com/arti-cles/2012/02/which-way-go-ce-mark-or-fda-approval. Accessed 21 July 2015.

12. FDA. Unsafe and ineffective devices approved in the EU that were not approved in the US. http://www.elsevierbi.com/~/media/Supporting%20Documents/The%20 Gray%20Sheet/38/20/FDA_EU_Devices_Report.pdf. Accessed 19 July 2015.

13. Paddock C. FDA panel conflict of interest restrictions too stringent say senators. http://www.medicalnewstoday.com/articles/235975.php. Accessed 22 July 2015.

14. Talamini MA. Benefit-risk paradigm for clinical trial design of obesity devices: FDA proposal. Surg Endosc. 2013;27(3):701. doi:10.1007/s00464-012-2726-1. Epub 2013 Jan 24.

15. Lerner H, Whang J, Nipper R. Benefit-risk paradigm for clinical trial design of obesity devices: FDA proposal. Surg Endosc. 2013;27(3):702–7. doi:10.1007/s00464-012-2724-3. Epub 2012 Dec 18.

8. Getting an Idea from Paper to Patient

Raymond P. Onders

This book begins with an introduction to some impressive surgical innovations that all began with an idea. Almost all surgical innovations begin with an idea on how to improve surgical care and not how to make a profit. As surgeons, we always put the need of the patients first, and our innovations also should do that. Throughout this book there are outlines of the regulatory requirements needed for use of a device in the human, so this chapter will not go into great depth in that area. The goal is to outline some of the steps needed when a surgeon has that "ah-ha" moment. Most of what I will be discussing will be based on my own two-decade odyssey with the development of a functional electrical device with surgically placed electrodes on the diaphragm (Diaphragm Pacing or DP) to improve respiration in multiple disease entities such as spinal cord injury (SCI) and amyotrophic lateral sclerosis (ALS) [1–3].

This chapter will simplify this process into four areas that are the keys to surgical innovation for medical devices: Personal Capabilities and Fortitude, Patents and Intellectual Property, Engineering and Development of Prototypes, and Business Development.

Personal Capabilities and Fortitude

A surgical idea usually begins when we are interacting with a patient and realize there should be a better way to help this patient, a simpler way to do this operation, a less painful way to do the operation, or a faster way to do this procedure to save anesthesia time for the patient. At times these ideas surface when we are telling the patient we have nothing to offer. Surgeons have the intellectual capability to consider

© Springer International Publishing Switzerland 2016
S.C. Stain et al. (eds.), *The SAGES Manual Ethics of Surgical Innovation*, DOI 10.1007/978-3-319-27663-2_8

different options but many times they do not have the time resources to maintain the focus and passion to oversee what will become a long-term project. I have now spent 18 years on my research and business development with the diaphragm pacing project. In the last decade alone, since the founding of the company Synapse Biomedical to commercialize diaphragm pacing, I have traveled over 800 days and over 1 million miles. Surgical innovators have to realize it takes time and effort.

Surgeons have to realize and understand that there may be financial risks in developing devices. I also did not realize when we took on the founding of this company what the financial implications were. I had no idea how much money is required to get a device to market. To date, I have been involved in spending over 25 million dollars to obtain FDA approval to allow patients access to the diaphragm pacing technology. I have learned how to raise money from venture capitalists, and I unfortunately learned how to weather the instability of the marketplace. In 2008, we received FDA approval for diaphragm pacing for spinal cord injured patients, were nearing the end of our trial in ALS, and our future looked bright. We were about to successfully raise additional funds to fast track this technology and begin research into using diaphragm pacing to decrease ventilator days in the intensive care units. Then the markets collapsed. Synapse Biomedical was running out of money and there was no available capital. To continue to provide diaphragm pacing that is life changing in SCI, we had to slow down our expansion to other diseases. This mandated layoffs of over half of the company. The company now did not have enough band width to do multiple projects at once. As a board member of Synapse Biomedical, I take to heart the fiduciary responsibility not only to shareholders but to the patients that use this technology. All surgeon inventors should maintain the safety of our patients even if it means slowing down the process.

One other barrier of innovation is the assumption of conflict of interest when developing devices. Conflict of interest should not limit your research but one needs to make sure everyone is notified of the conflict, including both patients and colleagues. Independent analysis of data is mandatory, and having other researchers and institutions duplicate the data does increase cost, but again will confirm safety and reproducibility.

Patents and Intellectual Property

When you have an idea, the first thing to do is go to what replaces the old library – the Internet – and "google it". Significant background internet research should be done before even discussing your idea with anyone else. All relevant medical articles should be researched to see if anyone else has already tried this and failed. Background information about the disease or condition should be analyzed. It is well described that failed innovations or research usually do not get published. A search on clinicaltrials.gov using the disease your idea is about may show some early human work being done that is similar to your idea. After our second successful patient in diaphragm pacing for spinal cord injury, who happened to be Christopher Reeve (Superman), I was asked on national television if this would work in ALS. In analyzing other researchers work in functional electrical stimulation of the extremities done a decade earlier in Japan for patients with ALS, their conclusion was that electrical stimulation did not improve survival or function but it did increase muscle mass [4]. Our conclusion of this study was that it was not a negative study, but that they were stimulating the wrong muscle – they could not stimulate the diaphragm. Diaphragm failure leads to respiratory failure and subsequent death in ALS; perhaps stimulating the diaphragm could alter that mode of death. That led us to the initial pilot trials and subsequent FDA approval for diaphragm pacing in a subgroup of ALS patients [5].

The other key entity to research is the US patent office website. You should search to see if someone or some entity has already thought of your idea. Most patents have diagrams so these should be reviewed to see if someone has already diagramed what you were contemplating. This search should be exhaustively done by yourself prior to "employing" anyone to help this. Once you believe that your idea is new, then you should protect it. Some altruistic physicians would say I will just publish it and let everyone know about it. This sounds great, but because of the cost of getting an idea through the regulatory hurdles; if it is not protected no company will ever build it because any other company could then build it after it is approved and they would lose their investment. The diaphragm electrodes that we use in pacing are great electrodes but a description of the electrode was unfortunately published prior to obtaining any intellectual property (IP) when the electrodes were first developed at my university by engineering students. Fortunately the manufacturing knows how and the applications of the electrodes have all been protected, but ideally it would have been best to have IP on the electrodes.

If you found that someone has a patent on your idea or is doing some preliminary human research, it would be imperative to reach out to the person or entity. Your initial idea was most likely to help patients and perhaps you could become the surgical champion of this idea even if someone else patented it first. Some ideas or patents are purely the result of patent mills that do not have true patient interests as their basis. If you believe this is the case, you could still help in the studies to provide this technology to patients.

If you have now identified that you have a new idea, the next step is to protect it. You should document the birthday of your idea by dating and notarizing the document. If you work in a university or employed by a medical center, you will realize that you only own part of your idea. The IP is most likely owned by these entities; since the 1990s, they all have technology transfer offices that will review your idea and should help with the provisional patent. This begins the process of protecting your idea. This can also be done by yourself at minimal cost. The conversion of the provisional patent to a full patent will require a patent attorney with experience in medical devices to make sure all of the appropriate claims are made. In my own case of diaphragm pacing for ALS, the time from provisional patent to full patent took 6 years with a trip for an in-person interview at the US patent office. My patent costs and attorney fees for all diaphragm pacing IP to date is well over a million dollars. This is just the beginning of the costs from an idea to the patient.

Engineering and Development of Prototypes

With the advent of 3D printing, rapid prototype manufacturing can create the device. This may even allow simulation in the constructed human anatomy. However, engineering the prototype will usually require partnering with engineers or engineering students if available. Before discussing your idea with others, a non-disclosure agreements (NDA) should be agreed to, especially if patent applications have not been filed. Depending on materials, the innovation may require biocompatible testing and corroborating evidence in animals. If this is needed, the complex standards of Good Laboratory Practices (GLP) will need to be followed. If the early studies do not follow these standards, the data cannot be used in FDA applications for future studies. It is important to identify engineering problems early in the development cycle and prevent their negative impact on a project. You do not want to repeat your initial animal studies, so very close collaboration with between the clinician and engineering is paramount.

Also, Good Manufacturing Practices (GMPs) have to be followed so that a device could be used in a first-in-human trial. This requires a manufacturer of record for the device. This was one of the initial reasons that Synapse Biomedical was founded. The entire device was constructed in our research lab for the first implant in 2000, but with changes in FDA regulations we needed a manufacturer of record to safely and reliably provide the device. Fortunately, there are only 300–500 new ventilator dependent spinal cord injured patients a year in the United States. Unfortunately, this is not an economic model that any company wants to enter into, I was unable to convince any available medical device companies to build the diaphragm pacing device. In order to provide this for patients we had to found our own company – Synapse Biomedical; which leads to the next section of this chapter.

Business Development

Early on in the development of a device, there has to be a market analysis of how the device would be used in practice. This also involves analysis of the FDA pathway for approval with an understanding of the differences in the average cost of approval. If it is a new Class III medical device that will require a full premarket approval (PMA), then the average costs will be 94 million dollars. If the device is close enough to an existing medical technology, then it may be approved through the 510k pathway which averages only 31 million dollars [6, 7]. The market for the device will have to be large enough to support the approval process if it is a low priced device or can it command a large price for a much smaller market. This involves development of a business plan which would outline costs of the regulatory burden, market analysis, and a perspective on the returns on investment. If this analysis looks promising then the next major decision for the innovator is to establish their own business or to license the technology to existing companies.

This is the time when most surgical innovators have already partnered with a management team. As much as we think that we, the clinical innovators, can do this ourselves, it is very difficult to understand all aspects of financing to partake this without help. The choice of your management team should be people that have your same moral and ethical obligations to the patient that would be using your device. They should not just be motivated by profit. This will be a long process so you should be compatible with them. They should have experience and understanding of the necessary regulatory, engineering and marketing areas of your device. This is the time when all innovators also realize that their percentage of the business will only go down. Hopefully the value will always go up, but one has to remember that there are always many failed devices. The amount of capital needed to get a product to market far exceeds your own capabilities, and therefore you have to accept that much of your ownership will be lost. This is when investment entities will place a value on your business; most of the time it will be less than what you believe your "sweat equity" is worth. As part of the fortitude of being an innovator you have to be willing to accept outside valuations of your device.

There are growing limitations to surgical innovations that include: an academic climate focusing on clinical productivity with a little protected research time; decreased corporate research funding from the affordable care act device tax burden; decreased private equity capital investment of $20 billion from 2011 to 2013; difficult coding and decreased reimbursement from insurance agencies; and the FDA regulatory burden [8, 9]. This will affect the ability to raise the capital necessary to allow a device to reach the market. However, if a device will help the patient and will decrease costs, then one will be able to find partners to get the innovation to market.

Conclusions

Surgical innovation is a never-ending process. During the process of developing your device and in analyzing your results, applications may change that can modify your business plans and markets. In my own research endeavor, diaphragm pacing went from a simple bypass of an injured spinal cord with diaphragm pacing to provide ventilation, to a device that overcomes newly found instability of respiration in ALS and ICU patients. ALS patients develop an instability of respiration that is based in our brainstem's "breathing center", which involves the lateral medulla and the pre-Botzinger complex [10].

Because of simultaneous experience in our spinal cord–injured patients receiving diaphragm pacing, we identified a group of patients who were implanted with DP and who recovered their ability to breath. We showed that these patients also developed an instability of respiration and control of breathing that required tracheostomy mechanical ventilation. After we implanted DP and freed them from the ventilator, they recovered their own control of ventilation and the DP wires were easily pulled out percutaneously [11]. The functional electrical stimulation of DP helped in the neuroplasticity and recovery of respiratory pathways. DP can induce changes in our brainstem and our automatic control of breathing, which became an additional application of our device. Innovators have to always continue to analyze their data for possible new applications or to see if there is no positive effect.

My initial research goals of a simple stable bypass of control of diaphragm function with electrodes are actually having much greater effects on the instability of respiratory control. This has also become the central piece of our present temporary use of DP in the ICU to help decrease the amount of time patients are on ventilators and hopefully decrease the greater than 100,000 tracheostomies done in the USA for failure to wean from ventilators. We have shown that DP can allow weaning from positive pressure ventilation when they have unilateral or bilateral diaphragm dysfunction [12]. With this growing data, a multicenter prospective trial would be needed to confirm this hypothesis. This means further intellectual property, engineering, capital raising and FDA discussions once again. Innovations always go back to this basic plan for each iteration of a device.

So after 18 years on this diaphragm pacing project, I realize there is no such thing as complete stability of surgical innovation. There is a stability of our surgical ethics – always do what is right for the patients; therefore, surgeons can and must innovate. We have the passion, and we know what our patient's clinical needs are. Always partner with people you enjoy being with because it will be a long road. Always maintain your respect for the patients, and do not be overcome by looking at finances first. Identify products and devices that work. Even if you are not the initial innovator, be involved in post-approval monitoring of new devices. We need to help our patients both with identifying products that work, but with identifying when innovations don't work.

Conflict of Interest Disclosure

Dr. Raymond Onders, University Hospitals of Cleveland and Case Western Reserve University School of Medicine have intellectual property rights involved with the diaphragm pacing system and equity in Synapse Biomedical who manufactures the device.

References

1. Onders RP, Aiyar H, Mortimer JT. Characterization of the human diaphragm muscle with respect to the phrenic nerve motor points for diaphragmatic pacing. Am Surg. 2004;70:241–7.
2. Onders RP, Ignagni AI, DeMarco AF, Mortimer JT. The learning curve of investigational surgery: lessons learned from the first series of laparoscopic diaphragm pacing for chronic ventilator dependence. Surg Endosc. 2005;19:633–7.
3. Onders R. The diaphragm how it affect my life and my career. The search for stability when the problem is instability. Am J Surg. 2015;2092(3):431–5.
4. Handa I, Matsushito N, Ihashi K, et al. A clinical trial of therapeutic electrical stimulation for amyotrophic lateral sclerosis. Tohoku J Exp Med. 1995;175:123–34.
5. Onders R, Elmo M, Kaplan C, Katirji B, Schilz R. Final analysis of the pilot trial of diaphragm pacing in amyotrophic lateral sclerosis with long term follow-up: diaphragm pacing positively affects diaphragm respiration. Am J Surg. 2014;207:393–7.
6. Naghshineh N, Brown S, Cederna PS, et al. Demystifying the US Food and Drug Administration: understanding regulatory pathways. Plast Reconstr Surg. 2014;134:559–69.
7. Sastry A. Overview of the US FDA medical device approval process. Curr Cardiol Resp. 2014;16:494.
8. Bergsland J, Elle OJ, Fosse E. Barriers to medical device innovation. Med Dev Evid Res. 2014;7:205–9.
9. Atlas SW. ObamaCare's anti-innovation effect. Wall Street J. 2014:1.
10. Onders R, Elmo MJ, Kaplan C, Katirji B, Schilz R. Identification of unexpected respiratory abnormalities in patients with amyotrophic lateral sclerosis through electromyographic analysis using intramuscular electrodes implanted for therapeutic diaphragmatic pacing. Am J Surg. 2015;209(3):451–6.
11. Posluszny JA, Onders R, Kerwin AJ, et al. Multicenter review of diaphragm pacing in spinal cord injury: successful not only in weaning from ventilators but also in bridging to independent respiration. J Trauma Acute Care Surg. 2014;76:303–10.
12. Onders R, Elmo MJ, Kaplan C, Katirji B, Schilz R. Extended Use of diaphragm pacing in patients with unilateral of bilateral diaphragm dysfunction: a new therapeutic option. Surgery. 2014;156:772–86.

9. How and Why Work with an Industry Partner?

Maria S. Altieri, Caitlin Halbert, and Aurora Pryor

Most device related advances in surgical care have arisen from partnerships between clinicians and their industry partners. These collaborations have led to benefits in imaging, minimal invasive techniques, and novel devices. This has allowed the surgeon to minimize complications and negative effects on quality of life following surgery, leading to improvement in patient outcomes [1]. These advances would not be possible without the merging of physician clinical expertise and the skills, knowledge and resources of engineers, businessmen, and other technical experts. Recently the interface between clinician and industry has come under fire through multiple avenues. Although scrutinized, this partnership is vital and drives innovation.

How Can I Work with Industry?

Corporate partners often recruit physicians as consultants in research, development, or marketing of devices and products [2, 3]. These relationships are critical to develop new devices or improve products in a clinically relevant way. Without clinical knowledge, engineers may develop products without true practical application. Prototype testing and improvement is also best accomplished with clinician input to make an end product that is easy to use and beneficial to patients. Without this clinical input, our industry partners would invest both time and money in a less efficient way and potentially develop products that were not appealing to surgeons.

© Springer International Publishing Switzerland 2016
S.C. Stain et al. (eds.), *The SAGES Manual Ethics
of Surgical Innovation*, DOI 10.1007/978-3-319-27663-2_9

Surgeons can also be innovators. Many new products available today were conceived by clinicians with or without industry involvement. It is very difficult, however, for a practicing surgeon to devote the necessary time and resources to carry a new product from concept to clinical use. In these situations, surgeons often reach out to either smaller idea incubators or larger device companies to help carry the product through the patent and prototype process through FDA approval, manufacturing, and distribution. Without these mutually beneficial relationships, many products would not make it into clinical use.

Physicians can also receive industry support for speaking at educational events. These relationships have the benefit of sharing new ideas and techniques with other surgeons. The physician can receive an honorarium for speaking, consulting, or teaching; have ownership interest in a product or device; receive a salary, royalties, or consulting fee; receive a research, fellowship, or lab support.

In 2007, an article in the New England Journal of Medicine reported that 28 % of department chairs received payments for consulting, talks, or enrolling patients in trials [2]. A more recent study published in 2010 showed that 18.3 % of physicians reported receiving reimbursements and 14.1 % received payments for professional services by industry [4]. These mechanisms required surgeons to disclose relationships, but there was no mechanism to verify the validity of their reporting. The Physician Payments Sunshine Act (PPSA) was enacted as part of the 2010 Affordable Care Act (ACA) [5]. This new policy requires industry partners the collect and publicly release information about physician-industry financial ties. The first collected data was published online in September of 2014. This policy will increase transparency in physician-industry relationships, but will it affect collaboration?

Why Work with Industry?

Collaboration between physicians and industry plays an integral part in surgical innovation. When entering an operating room one can witness many examples of how industry has played a role in the advancement of surgery. The most obvious role of industry is the ability to fund, develop, and implement technological surgical innovations more efficiently than an individual or an institution without industry support. A study showed that nearly one in five patented devices was invented by a physician or with the participation of physicians. Orthopedic surgeons, general surgeons, and cardiologists hold the majority of the patented inventions. Physicians who invent new devices are typically not involved in the manufacturing or marketing of the product, as the majority lack the business and regulatory knowledge [6]. Thus, without such collaboration, many of these devices would not have come to market.

Industry partners also play an important role in research and education. The National Institutes of Health has historically been a primary sponsor of research in the USA. However, with tightening government budgets, industry is an alternative source for support [7]. Many research grants are funded by companies, in addition to opportunities such as investigator initiated studies (IIS), when investigators have been denied by the government and surgical societies for funding. These resources are often critical for young investigators to get started with research. These mechanisms can also provide seed funding for larger government-sponsored projects.

From an educational prospective, many companies have historically been involved in support for residency and fellowship training positions [7, 8]. For example, industry has sponsored many surgical fellowship-training positions in non-ACGME accredited fellowship programs. After the Foundation of Surgical Fellowships (FSF) was founded in 2010, direct industry-funded training fellowships have mostly become extinct, although industry support is the lifeblood of the FSF [9]. As industry support for fellowships dwindles, the future of post-graduate surgical education is potentially in jeopardy.

Although many surgeons consider industry support only for non-Continuing Medical Education (CME) courses, CME is another area that has received support from industry [10]. Most society meetings are largely dependent on industry sponsorships. Without industry support, we would not be able to provide high-level educational experiences for surgeons. As industry support is questioned, the future of surgical meetings may be in jeopardy. Companies are vital in educating physicians about new devices and procedures, and staying current with surgical care.

How Deal with Conflict of Interest?

Definition of COI

There are clearly benefits from the collaboration between physicians and industry. However, there is also a growing concern that such a relationship may influence a surgeon's professional judgment. The public is concerned that physicians may place financial benefits ahead of patients' welfare when making clinical decisions. As such, the term Conflict of Interest (COI) has been coined to describe a set of circumstances that creates a risk that professional judgment or actions can be unduly influenced by a secondary interest, either monetary or some other kind of personal gain. Proponents of disclosure of COI state that it is important to ensure integrity of professional judgment and patient trust. Critics cite that disclosures may hinder productive research and innovation [11].

Concerns Regarding Industry-Physician Cooperation

Financial ties between physicians and pharmaceutical companies are extensive and controversial. The concerns regarding industry-physician partnership come from the notion that people generally tend to reciprocate, i.e. people generally feel obliged to return favors. In the past, companies have enticed physicians with free lunches, pens, etc. Many had concerns that no-matter how small these gifts are, physicians will try to reciprocate. In addition, it was feared that physicians can also be influenced by advertisements from companies. In 1992, an article regarding physician drug-prescribing trends before and following drug company-sponsored symposiums were examined regarding two drugs. It was determined that following symposiums both medications were prescribed significantly higher, vouching for the effect of drug companies on physicians [12].

A recent study evaluated the perception of the US population regarding various industry ties with physicians. Interestingly, findings showed that the general population was more influenced by payment type rather than payment amount. Specifically, the US population was more critical of physicians who owned stocks in certain companies rather than receiving payments. Further, the survey showed that the general public was more approving of physicians receiving free drug samples and consulting fees. Finally, physicians that had no financial ties were perceived as honest, but inexperienced [13].

Inappropriate Physician-Industry Relationships

There are many examples where financial ties between physicians and industry, and even medical associations and industry have been inappropriate. The majority of these involve failure to disclose COIs.

A great example of how failure to provide full disclosure can be perceived as impropriety is the story of Dr. Jay Yadav. Dr. Yadav was the chair of Cleveland Clinic Foundation Innovations, who was dismissed from his post in 2005. The events that lead to his dismissal were centered on his failure to disclose the fact that he was receiving a 1 % royalty fee from the sale of AngioGuard devices (Cordis/Johnson & Johnson). Dr. Yadav invented the device and subsequently sold it to the company in 1999. He had initiated the SAPPHIRE trial, which included the device. His royalty payments were directly tied to the success of the device for which he was performing the clinical trial. In addition, he did not disclose his conflict of interest to several medical journal articles, which mentioned the device. Although Dr. Yadav did not think he had conflict of interest, his behavior was regarded as inappropriate and led to his dismissal [14]. It is generally considered inappropriate to do clinical trials if the investigator has significant financial ties to the product being tested.

Individual physicians are not the only ones that have been accused of impropriety. Various companies have been exposed to provide excessive incentives to physicians. More recently, GlaxoSmithKline was under scrutiny and was ordered to pay $3 billion dollars for questionable practices regarding off-label uses of a medication. The investigation revealed that the company spent lavish amounts for physician-associated incentives for the use of their product [15]. In light of such occurrences, transparency is vital in order to keep public's trust in medicine, ensure patient's welfare, and the quality of medical education.

Transparency

Although lacking empirical evidence, the strategy of addressing potential conflict of interest is the enhancement and enforcement of disclosures by physicians, also known as transparency [16]. As mentioned above, due to growing public concerns, in 2007, a new federal legislation called The Physicians Payment Sunshine Act of 2007 was proposed. Although it initially was not enacted, it became official in 2010 as part of the Patient Protection and Affordable Care Act [5]. This has led to companies publicly releasing details of the payments made to physicians and other professionals for any interaction including, dinners, talks, research, and consulting [17]. The database can be accessed at https://openpaymentsdata.cms.gov/.

What Does Sages Do?

As the need for structure and oversight has become evident, organizations such as the Society of American Gastrointestinal and Endoscopic Surgeons (SAGES) and American College of Surgeons (ACS) have been on the forefront by providing surgeons with guidelines to help innovation in a structured way. The major tasks are to help assist introduction of new technology and techniques without hindering progress.

In 2010, the SAGES Industry Relations Task Force released their statement on the relationship between professional medical associations (PMAs) and industry. The paper states that the collaboration between PMAs and physicians is indeed integral to the process of development and deployment of new medications, tools, and procedures. This is especially true in the area of surgery. It further highlights four points: the medical device industry is different from the pharmaceutical industry in the approach to the development of new products; medical device development industry is essential to physician innovation and development of new technology; research and development and education must be separated from sales and marketing; full disclosure and complete transparency of physician financial relationships with industry are critical [18].

Conclusion

Collaboration between industry and physicians is vital for innovation. These relationships benefits surgeons, patients, and/or industry partners. In order to avoid scrutiny and to have an efficient partnership, transparency and full disclosures are important for such relationships to be efficient.

References

1. Barker CF, Kaiser LR. Is surgical science dead? The excelsior Society lecture. J Am Coll Surg. 2004;198:1–19.
2. Campbell EG, Gruen RL, Mountford J, Miller LG, Cleary PD, Blumenthal D. A national survey of physician-industry relationships. N Engl J Med. 2007;356(17): 1742–50.
3. Lo B, Field MJ, eds. Conflict of interest in medical research, education, and practice. Washington, DC: The National Academies Press; 2009. Robertson C, Rose S,

Kesselheim AS. Effect of financial relationships on the behaviors of health care professionals: a review of the evidence. J Law Med Ethics. 2012;40(3):452–66.

4. Campbell EG, Rao SR, DesRoches CM, Iezzoni LI, Vogeli C, Bolcic-Jankovic D, Miralles PD. Physician professionalism and changes in physician-industry relationships from 2004 to 2009. Arch Intern Med. 2010;170:20.

5. Mackey TK, Liang BA. Physician payment disclosure under health care reform: will the Sun shine? J Am Board Fam Med. 2014;26(3):327–31.

6. Chatterji AK, Fabrizio KR, Mitchell W, Schulman KA. Physician-industry cooperation in the medical device industry. Health Aff (Millwood). 2008;27(6):1532–43.

7. Dorsey ER, de Roulet J, Thompson JP, Reminick JI, Thai A, White-Stellato Z, Beck CA, George BP, Moses 3rd H. Funding of US biomedical research, 2003–2008. JAMA. 2010;303(2):137–43.

8. Kuehn BM. Pharmaceutical industry funding for residencies sparks controversy. JAMA. 2005;293:1572–80.

9. http://www.surgicaleducation.com/research-fellowship-serf. The Association of Surgical Education.

10. 2006–2007. Accreditation Council for Graduate Medical Education. ACGME Annual Report Data.

11. Sade RM. Full disclosure: where is the evidence for nefarious conflicts of interest? Ann Thorac Surg. 2011;92(2):417–20.

12. Orlowski L, Wateska JP. The effects of pharmaceutical firm enticements on physician prescribing patterns. There's no such thing as a free lunch. Chest. 1992;102(1):270–3.

13. Perry JE, Cox D, Cox AD. Trust and transparency: patient perceptions of physicians' financial relationships with pharmaceutical companies. J Law Med Ethics. 2014;42(4):475–91.

14. Wood S. Cleveland Clinic fires Dr Jay Yadav for undisclosed conflicts of interest Shelley Wood. Medscape, 2006. http://www.medscape.com/viewarticle/788663. Accessed 17 Mar 2015.

15. Lee W, Rocke D, Holsinger C. Surgical innovation, industry partnership, and the enemy within. Head Neck. 2014;34(4):461–5.

16. Katz D, Caplan AL, Merz JF. All gifts large and small: toward an understanding of the ethics of pharmaceutical industry gift-giving. Am J Bioeth. 2003;3:39–46.

17. Propublica. Dollars for Docs. How industry dollars reach your doctors. https://projects.propublica.org/docdollars/. Accessed 2 Apr 2015.

18. Surgeons, Society of American Gastrointestinal and Endoscopic. Society of American Gastrointestinal and Endoscopic Surgeons(SAGES)statement on the relationship between professional medical associations and industry. Surg Endosc. 2010;24(4):742–4.

10. Status and Impact of Evolving Medical Device Venture Capital Landscape on Innovation

Richard S. Stack, William N. Starling, Mudit K. Jain, and James Melton

Innovation in medical devices, and the subsequent health improvements they generate, predominantly comes from inventors, most often located in academia or small development firms. For these innovative devices to have their intended impact on human health, they must be fully developed, adequately tested, and made accessible to patients, while generating sufficient returns for their developers to grow and for their investors to generate attractive returns for this high-risk capital. These steps receive support mostly in the form of venture capital. Without such capital, important gains in the treatment of health problems decline. It is also important to note the value of the medtech industry to the economy. The US Department of Commerce reports that the US medical device market, currently the largest in the world, stands at $110 billion and is slated to grow to $133 billion by 2016. This is an estimated 38 % of the global marketplace. In the USA alone, there are an estimated 6,500 medical device companies, 80 % of which employ less than 50 people [1]. A healthy medtech industry carries substantial benefits to patients, the public health, and the overall economy. The enabling investments in these companies warrant attention. The status of such investments, their structure, and their impact on innovation in the medical device arena has changed in recent years, necessitating changes in the way innovators, investors, and their companies approach their efforts.

Venture capital is typically defined as high-risk capital made available to small businesses, usually startups, which do not have ready access to other sources of capital, yet offer substantial growth potential over time. For various reasons explained below and the complex nature

© Springer International Publishing Switzerland 2016   89
S.C. Stain et al. (eds.), *The SAGES Manual Ethics*
of Surgical Innovation, DOI 10.1007/978-3-319-27663-2_10

of such innovation, these firms present high risk for investors as well as the possibility of high returns. While many medical device/technology firms are started with grants or individual investments (i.e., friends and family, angel investors, etc.), they soon need significant capital where traditional borrowing is not possible due to lack of revenues, short operating history, or insufficient collateral. However, early stage capital needs are most often below the minimums set for institutional investors and larger credit companies, and the companies themselves are viewed as too risky. In addition, venture capital investments often bring technical and management expertise. These resources are invaluable in many cases and outside the capabilities of the start-up company.

While venture capital is at times the only source of capital to new companies, founders must recognize that venture investors typically participate in company decisions and policies, and they own equity. This arrangement can be seen as invasive, or at least cumbersome, to some entrepreneurs.

Development of new, meaningful ideas is a challenging proposition, especially in light of the hurdles that exist between concept and commercial acceptance. Many of the areas involved are unpredictable and uncertain, and often beyond the control of the entrepreneurs. These hurdles, coupled with the time and resources needed to overcome them, underlie the risks faced by medical device companies and their venture capitalists partners. The detailed challenges faced and trends in each area are explored further in this chapter.

With respect to how the venture investment process usually works, five steps normally occur:

1. Venture Capital Fundraising. In a venture capital fund, the capital is raised from investors who become part of a limited partnership. Members are most often high net worth individuals, pension funds, insurance companies, endowments, foundations, and other pools of capital created by like-minded parties for investment purposes. Lately, corporations, philanthropic organizations, and patient advocacy groups have become more significant investors both through their own funds and participation in funds created by more traditional means. In each case, the partnership defines what types of investments will be made with accumulated capital, bounds on the size of individual investments, the phase of the companies supported, and the time frame or lifespan over which the fund will exist.

2. Investment. Once the fund is closed, its management team finds companies of interest, conducts diligence, and enters into deals.

These investments are often referred to as "portfolio companies." Funds are most often put into the identified firms at predetermined milestones and during various "rounds."

3. Growth and Management of Portfolio Company. The venture firm will often participate directly in a number of ways, mostly related to corporate policy and strategy, bring specific knowledge of use to the firm, and introduce potential partners, customers, and other contributors to the firm, and by membership on the Board of Directors.

4. Exit. With success, a typical investment will advance to the point of an IPO or acquisition in 5–10 years as a way of garnering substantial capital for continued operation and growth. This is the most substantial method for investors to achieve a return on their investment.

5. Return. Upon an exit, investors receive funds based on their relative ownership. These funds are then available for reinvestment in new opportunities as the cycle of development and growth continues [2].

The decision to invest in a given company involves multiple criteria including clinical needs, technical/scientific variables, market factors, business model, regulatory challenges, legal issues (especially around intellectual property), reimbursement, market acceptance, timing, and the management team involved. These items are discussed in detail later in the chapter. However, it is useful to discuss the recent history of venture capital support of medical device innovation and the implications of recent trends on this arena.

Historical Position of Venture Capital in Medical Device Development

Historically, medical device development is highly dependent on venture funding. Over the past 20 years, venture investment in the USA has gone through two apparent cycles: one peaking in 2000 and the other, much smaller, peak occurring in 2007 as seen in Fig. 10.1. Though 2014 showed an uptick in overall venture funding in the USA, all of the increase occurred in the Technology/Computers/Telecom sector and the Life Sciences sector saw a marked turndown.

Except for some late year activity in 2014, venture capital has remained relatively flat in total and has dropped as a percentage of total financing. Table 10.1 details the areas where capital was raised from all sources since 2007. As the largest growth in capital raise occurred via debt, innovation likely faced new hurdles as debt can hamper a young

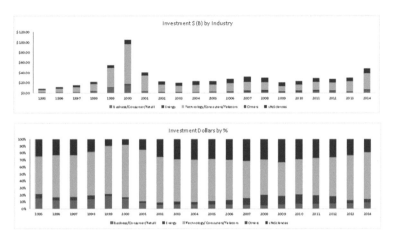

Fig. 10.1. Total investments by industry (US). (Data from the National Venture Capital Association).

Table 10.1. Capital raised in the USA and Europe (US $).

Type	2008	2009	2010	2011	2012	2013	2014
Venture	39 %	36 %	23 %	22 %	17 %	13 %	16 %
IPO	10 %	0 %	2 %	4 %	2 %	1 %	5 %
Follow-on and other	16 %	14 %	11 %	13 %	4 %	13 %	7 %
Debt	35 %	50 %	64 %	62 %	77 %	73 %	71 %
Total ($ million)	$1,311	$12,922	$20,820	$19,081	$26,023	$31,643	$27,306

Data from Ernst & Young, Pulse of the Industry, Medical Technology Report 2012

company's ability to raise additional capital, whether through venture capital or other vehicles.

Finally, when looking at the trend in the number of transactions executed as detailed in Fig. 10.2, the average number has been relatively flat over the last 10 years. With the total amount invested being slightly larger, there is the implication that certain, individual deals drive the average and that these deals are mostly later stage ones, that is, more mature companies.

More telling is the drop in venture capital support for medtech companies. As mentioned, these innovative companies are supported mostly by venture capital. The trends in the charts in Fig. 10.3 reflect

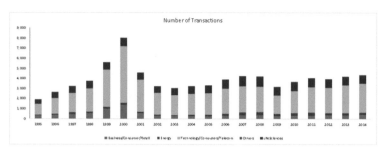

Fig. 10.2. Number of transactions. (Data from the National Venture Capital Association).

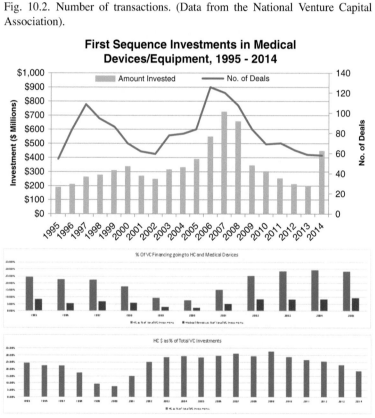

Fig. 10.3. Total investment in medical devices and equipment, 1995–2014. (Data from the National Venture Capital Association).

not only a decline in overall healthcare investment from the venture world, but a more rapid decline in the proportion of this funding taken in by medtech firms [3].

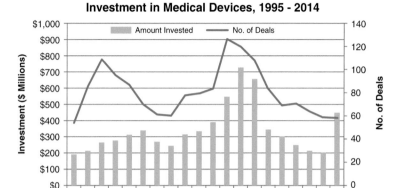

Fig. 10.4. First sequence investments in medical devices 1995–2014. (Data from The MoneyTree™ Report, PricewaterhouseCoopers and the National Venture Capital Association, 2015).

Finally, and potentially the most significant trend, Fig. 10.4 shows a precipitous drop in first sequence, venture investments in medical device development, both in terms of money and number of deals done. While there is an increase in 2014, this is likely due to a small number of large deals not typical for the last several years. As discussed, the lack of resources, especially from the source most likely to accept the risk-reward ratio involved, is a serious threat to the ability for this entire sector to bring new products to the market. In particular, fewer resources in the initial sequence stop new ideas from getting started.

According to PricewaterhouseCoopers, software, media and entertainment, and biotech garner the largest venture investments and this trend will continue [4]. Losing the battle with other sectors for capital amidst changing security regulations and tax codes is challenging enough for medtech enterprises. A number of other issues more specific to the medtech arena raise the level are of concern in the near future.

Medical Device Development

Life sciences as a whole may be the most complex investment area, facing downward trends as discussed. Overall, many factors are impacting the size, type, and source of venture funding such as movements to emerging markets, competition from new markets outside the USA and Europe, changing and often more demanding and cumbersome regulations, changing/unpredictable reimbursement policies, changing decision processes, and changing models for the way care is provided.

Medtech carries many of these complexities along with some specific items that hamper the investment needed to drive innovation. Closer scrutiny of a few specific items raise particular concern for future investments in medical device innovation, especially in the USA, which remains the largest market and source of such innovation, including:

1. Overall trends in costs and time needed to get to market and/or exit
2. Increased regulatory burden
3. Increased tax burdens
4. Increased reimbursement/payment challenges
5. Increased industry consolidation and
6. Interactions across technologies

Each of these warrants consideration as development plans are made and investments are placed. All have an impact on the risks associated with getting to market, the time and expense of doing so, and the eventual return generated. The combination of so many factors creates management challenges for innovators running new companies and a more complex risk profile for investors with the option of putting capital into other less complex endeavors.

Overall Trends in Costs and Time

Creating and marketing medical devices is a risky pursuit. The process from idea to practical clinical application is long and expensive. Traditionally, early research is performed in academic institutions, while device development, testing, and production occur in the corporate environment. Processes are costly and frequently take years to accomplish. In spite of extensive testing of products, product failures do occur after they reach the market, potentially causing serious medical problems for individuals and financial disaster for the manufacturer.

A 2010 study, out of Stanford University surveying about 20 % of all US medtech companies, estimates that the average cost of taking a 510(k) product from concept through clearance is $31 million. For the more complex PMA process, gaining approval costs approximately $94 million [4].

Depending on the complexity of the device involved and the size of the target patient population, the average development time for a 510(k) product to reach the market is 3–5 years, while one requiring the PMA process is 5–10 years.

These are large sums of money and long periods of time, especially considering the investments do not include the sales and marketing expenses necessary to launch the technologies, nor the cost to set up operations and manufacturing. These figures and timelines are to get the device through regulatory approval but not yet at the point where it starts earning revenue. Most investors and founders seek an exit, typically via acquisition or IPO, along the way to obtain their return earlier and not have to shoulder the burden of growing a market and supporting operations.

Increased Regulatory Burden

The Federal Drug Administration (FDA) oversees the approval process for new medical technologies sold in the USA, doing so under the two-fold responsibility of protecting public health and promoting innovation. Within the FDA, the Center for Devices and Radiological Health (CDRH) has the responsibility of reviewing applications for new medical devices. In recent years, after a number of notable safety issues and product recalls, FDA's emphasis has been more on patient safety than innovation.

With pressure from industry, investors and certain patient advocacy groups to improve regulatory review times and processes through added resources, Congress enacted legislation, first in 2003, then again in 2012 to create, and increase, user fees paid by industry applicants with their new product submissions. A review written jointly by the California Healthcare Institute and the Boston Consulting Group [5] pointed out that during the first phase of user fees, contrary to the intention, approval timelines actually increased, and that the more recent timeframe under higher fees shows some evidence of improvement, but there are insufficient data to confirm a lasting trend.

A number of studies have explored the issue of FDA approval timelines for medical devices, with specific comparison to medical device approvals made in Europe, the second largest market for such products. Two major differences in structure and approach between the USA and Europe exist that underlie the differences in how long it takes new devices to obtain approval. First, there is the difference in the type of evidence required. In the USA, FDA requires "safety and efficacy" proof for a PMA device and "substantial equivalence" for a 510(k) device, which also includes an element of effectiveness. In Europe, the burden of proof to obtain a CE Mark, the marketing and distribution approval, relates only to safety. Second, the review and approval process itself is handled very differently. In Europe, this process relies extensively on entities called Notified Bodies, which may be private companies or foundations. There are about 50 such entities accredited by the member states of the European Union, which gives them the ability to determine whether a product, a medical device in this instance, meets the predefined standards of the EU Medical Devices Directive. If a positive determination results, then the company can obtain a CE Mark. These entities therefore offer numerous avenues for review versus the single, centralized agency in the USA, FDA's CDRH. While the differing structures do not guarantee differences in development timelines and costs, they certainly lay a foundation for different results.

In fact, significant differences have been found. The Stanford study pointed out that greater than 75 % of the development costs for a new medical device in the USA involve regulatory-related activities ($24 out of $31 million for a 510(k) device and $75 out of $94 million for a PMA device). The study also found significantly longer timelines for approval in the USA (510(k) and PMA applications) compared to those in Europe (CE Mark) (Table 10.2).

The additional 2–4 years that a device may take to obtain clearance in the USA is costly in multiple directions. By taking more time to get to market, more money is spent, time under patent coverage is spent, market

Table 10.2. 510(k) and PMA regulatory timelines.

	FDA reported review time	**US companies' experience in the USA**	**US companies' experience in Europe**
501(k)	Average time from receipt to final decision = 3 months	Average time from first filing to clearance = 10 months/ Average time from first communication to clearance = 31 months	Average time from first communication to certificate = 7 months
PMA	Average time from filing to approval on original PMA = 9 months	Average time from first communication to approval = 54 months	Average time from first communication to certificate = 11 months

Data from FDA Impact on US Medical Technology Innovation: A Survey of Over 200 Medical Technology Companies, J. Makower et. al. for Stanford University, MDMA, NVCA, and PricewaterhouseCoopers, LLP, pg 22 conditions change, and patients continue to go without a new therapy. As the FDA requires more evidence, this time is more costly still.

While the FDA may have a different structure than other agencies abroad, particularly those in Europe, it appears a considerable part of the gap in approval times and the consequential impact on investments, company values, and patient access is due to the manner in which the FDA interacts with applicant companies. More data from the Stanford Study reflect difficulties in dealing with the FDA. Across the areas of predictability, reasonableness, transparency, and overall experience consistently rated their experience dealing with the CE Mark process much more favorably than their experience with the FDA (Fig. 10.5).

Though these areas are difficult to quantify, the consistency of responses and the significant differences demonstrate a clear perception by companies that the FDA is less predictable, reasonable, and transparent than their European counterparts. Small start-up companies launching new technologies often have limited capabilities to negotiate regulatory issues. Coupled with limited financial resources, uncertainty as to the path they take and the expectations of those that determine their fate with respect to approval to market their product is a young company's worst nightmare. Consequently, it is predictable to see how an environ-

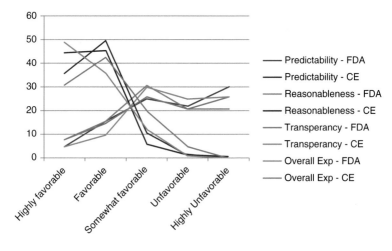

Fig. 10.5. Company ratings of FDA and EU regulatory interactions. (Data from FDA Impact on US Medical Technology Innovation: A Survey of Over 200 Medical Technology Companies, J. Makower et. al. for Stanford University, MDMA, NVCA, and PricewaterhouseCoopers, LLP).

ment with additional data requirements and unknown or changing expectations can lead to delays, additional costs, and lower investor interest. The outcome often becomes less innovation developed in the USA for US patients.

Increased Tax Burden

Two tax issues impact the economics of medical device innovation in the USA in important ways and with implications beyond the profitability of a given firm. One is general and one is very specific for this sector. The general item relates to the US statutory corporate tax rate, which stands at 39.1 % (a combination of a 35 % federal rate and the average state level rate), one of, if not the highest in the world. In comparison, the average rate in Europe is 18.6 %, and in a few countries around the world, it is 0 %. Also, the trend in most countries outside of the USA has been a decline in corporate tax rates, which encourages investment and growth in those locations [6, 7]. With deductions and other programs, the effective tax rate in the USA may be considerably lower. Such options exist in other countries as well, and the administrative burden of managing the accounting and filing complexities needed to achieve lower rates carries additional costs. As companies see high US tax rates as an increasingly negative issue for their bottom line, the logical step is to domicile their corporation in areas where tax rates are considerably lower, freeing up capital for growth and shareholder returns. The most notable move in this regard was the merger of Medtronic and Covidien, which resulted in the largest medical device company in the world forming its headquarters in Ireland. As more companies pursue this strategy, medical device innovation in the USA faces additional risk.

More specific to the medical device industry, in 2010 Congress enacted the Patient Protection and Affordable Care Act, which included a medical device excise tax of 2.3 % tax on medical device sales. For detailed language see:

- 26 USC 4191; Health Care and Education Reconciliation Act of 2010, Section 1405 (Public Law 111–152) [8].
- For purposes of the tax, a device is defined as intended for humans as defined in section 201(h) of the Federal Food, Drug and Cosmetic Act.
- Internal Revenue Service, Final Rule, Taxable Medical Devices, Dec. 7, 2012, 77 FR 72924 [9].

This tax is assessed without regard to profitability, placing a tremendous burden on young, early stage companies [10]. Ernst and Young estimate this to raise the effective tax rate for a medtech company by 29 %. The impact on after-tax profitability can be as high as 6.6 %, definitely a negative aspect for potential investors. The net effect of this tax on a "venture-financed, loss-making, young, start-up" is that expensive venture capital is paying the government taxes. This puts US venture-backed companies at a special disadvantage compared to other parts of the world where the governments are pouring money into venture funds to develop local industry.

The two leading trade organizations for this industry, the Medical Device Manufacturers Association [11, 12] and the Advanced Medical Technology Association [13], analyzed the impact of the excise tax, finding the following:

- 195,000 US jobs lost – 39,000 in the industry and 156,000 indirectly related jobs
- 53 % reduction in R&D investments by US medtech companies
- 75 % of companies postponed or canceled capital investments, new facilities, or new venture investments

    Also, these companies said a repeal of the excise tax would lead them to:

- Hire new employees (85 % of respondents)
- Increase R&D spending (80 % of respondents) on average by 14 %

A prominent consumer advocacy group, the Consumer Protection Union, formulated a different view of the medical device excise tax [11]. The organization's brief outlines three justifications for keeping the tax:

1. Shared contribution to cover new insured people
2. Bigger pool of covered/insured people to sell to
3. Industry is profitable

While the increased funding to broaden coverage dictated by the Affordable Care Act is an obvious need, there is no obvious reason why the medical device industry should be singled out in this regard. There is the argument that more people will have coverage, and therefore, the number of potential customers in need of, and capable of, paying for new medical devices increases. In reality, the need does not change and the potential reimbursement is questionable as there is no assurance that the new device will be covered. There is also extensive discussion concerning the profitability of the medical device industry, and the relatively minor, financial impact such a tax has on the growth and returns seen by these firms. However, the discussion itself points out that most of the high profit margins belong to the large, publically traded firms. In addition, the same discussion highlights the fact that the medical device industry is made up of many smaller firms, with their revenues and profits based on a single product, unlike other sectors within healthcare. As mentioned here, a sales tax is particularly hard on a smaller company, especially if it has not reached profitability. In many instances and in growing numbers, the very large medtech companies support development in smaller companies and later license the technology or acquire the smaller company. Here, they are essentially reinvesting their supposedly ultra-high profits back into innovation, which they can bring to market in a more expansive and effective manner.

Update: As discussed, the medical device excise tax enacted as part of the Affordable Care Act (IRS code section 4191) put a 2.3% tax on the revenues of medical device companies. However, The Consolidated Appropriation Act, 2016 (Pub. 6. 114-113) was signed into law December 18, 2015 providing for a two year moratorium on the excise tax. While this is a welcome development for the medtech industry, it still poses a bit of uncertainty as the 2 year period could end with no renewal, there could a permanent repeal of the tax, or there could be a string of extensions.

Increased Reimbursement Challenge

An important item to remember is that regulatory approval to market a medical device in the USA does not guaranteed coverage or payment for the device. Similar challenges apply in Europe and other jurisdictions. Once the regulatory hurdles mentioned earlier are cleared for a particular medical device, CMS, the agency that approves Medicare and Medicaid payments, must approve coverage of the device for the FDA-cleared indications under an independent process. There are also requirements for many new devices to demonstrate other, nonclinical, benefits such as resources utilization, cost savings, and reduced complications. Savvy companies collect much of these data during their clinical development, but uncertainties exist during that stage as to what data are pertinent for the later discussion. Some private payers have recently insisted that medical device companies show cost-benefit advantages to existing therapies in at least six peer-reviewed journals prior to making a coverage determination. Once coverage is granted, payment codes are generated. During the process, there are ongoing discussions with the company concerning value and pricing. Here again, there is considerable uncertainty as to the timelines for coverage and setting codes, and the price. This process can take 12–15 months, and in some cases up to 3 years following FDA approval.

Private payers typically follow CMS in their coverage and coding decisions, building on the foundation built by CMS but delaying the opportunity further for a new technology to get to patients.

Adding to the uncertainty are changes in the manner in which healthcare technologies are paid for in terms of their perceived value (and subsequently agreed-upon price) and who has the most influence in evaluation and purchasing decisions for new devices. Traditionally, physicians drove the selection of what treatment, and specifically which medical device, a patient received. In Ernst and Young's report [14], survey results present a picture of considerable change in the near future on such decisions. The report depicts the move by hospitals away from mere cost-cutting on specific items to more emphasis on broader elements of cost and care. Specifically, items such as reduced hospital stays, surgical efficiency, drug utilization, and readmissions are becoming more important.

Even the focus on broader cost management does not fully capture the direction foreseen by the survey participants. The perceived shift away from cost-cutting to value generation at the level of the hospital is driven in part by new legislation and other initiatives. Health care reform initiatives are more central in the planning and decision-making for hospitals, particularly in terms of the services and technologies they offer. Once again, medical device companies face an imprecise future, forecasted to require proof of value that is not currently well defined or captured. The criteria used for such assessments will continue to evolve, another type of uncertainty making it difficult for companies to plan well as they bring new devices to the market.

While the study also showed that price remains central to the discussion and the uptake of a new device, a shift from user-centric areas for product differentiation to quantifiable impact on patient outcomes and service delivery is the new paradigm. Products will have to use data to demonstrate clinical outcomes, show value to the system, and share risks.

The combination of these trends leads to a reduction in the influence of physicians in the selection of the devices offered and used. Going forward, the expectation is that those with budgeting and spending authority, that is, CFO, procurement, purchasing and payers, will play a larger role in such decisions. If that is indeed the case, the development of new devices will involve new data and its presentation to new decision-makers.

Increased Industry Consolidation

The recent Medtronic and Covidien merger (over \$46B and almost 2x larger than the next largest medtech deal) reflects a number of aspects of the corporate environment that pose new hurdles for the small, innovative medical device company. Such deals typically seek to bring cost savings through operational synergies, broader product offerings to create "1-stop shopping" model, and expanded distribution (typically to a global scale for large mergers). Recently, two additional trends have spurred consolidation of large firms. One is the corporate tax issue referenced above, where companies seek to protect profits that can be used to spur growth, development, and acquisitions. The other is the increase in divestitures (or spinouts) of certain divisions or product lines.

A small number of larger firms consolidate resources, intellectual capital, and access to the market. For those small, innovative companies looking to be acquired, or at least partner with a larger firm, there are fewer places to look and less of a competitive market for their offering as an acquisition. With increased divestitures, the acquirers themselves are putting competitive offerings into the field with mature operations. Once again, trends are difficult for a small firm with limited resources to address.

The contrasting opportunity may exist as mid-sized companies wishing to grow and compete acquire smaller firms rapidly.

Interactions Across Technologies

As discussed, the procurement environment is changing with different variables becoming more important and different people having more influence in purchasing decisions. Combining firms often means bringing multiple products together in the same sales effort. Even from a technological viewpoint, combining two or more devices, or devices with drugs, biologics, or services, may offer better, more coordinated care to patients and more efficiency to the system involved. While logic and opportunity may drive such combinations and product interactions, bundled technologies present increased complexity in terms of studying the collective effectiveness, gaining approval of the combination, managing relationships across multiple vendors, and marketing in a coordinated manner. Once again, the small, innovative medtech firm is faced with a more complex undertaking with a poorly defined path to success, and being highly dependent on products made and distributed by others.

The emergence of Accountable Care Organizations (ACOs) demonstrates one scenario where these issues all culminate. The decision-making is based on measures of quality of care and patient outcomes. Purchasing is done in a centralized manner. Selling to such organizations requires a sales and marketing enterprise beyond what is typical of small companies. It also points out the need for such caregivers to find, and optimally utilize, new technologies that combine improvement in patients' outcomes, process of care, and the economics of providing care.

Conclusions

In the USA, there are over 6,000 medical device companies in the USA where each faces multiple challenges:

- Decreasing capital from venture capital, the traditional source of enabling funds
- Increased international competition, both for technologies and for investment dollars
- Increased complexity in the marketplace
- Increased regulatory burdens in the USA
- Changing criteria in the methods by which new technologies are covered and reimbursed

Overcoming these challenges as a start-up, medical device company, no matter how innovative their technology may be, is impractical for many of these companies and their founders if traditional methods are used and trends of the last decade continue. Traditional venture capital support has leveled out, at best. For companies to thrive, they likely need new funding sources, niches where competition for resources is likely not as stiff, where partnerships readily present themselves, or where larger corporate players have a stronger and urgent need to add technologies to their portfolios. New opportunities exist in terms of looking at developing markets and new funding entities, but a lack of data about these areas makes forecasting risky and planning uncertain. The innovators of the future will need innovation beyond just their technology.

Recent Developments and Hope for the Future

While it appears many of the traditional, or "standard," methods of innovating and securing the necessary resources to create and develop new medical devices face significant challenges and negative trends, there are a number of trends that point to a more positive future.

New Markets

World markets are changing and as population and economic realities change, so do the markets for medical devices. The BRIC countries (Brazil, Russia, India, and China) make up 40 % of the world's demand for better healthcare technologies and quality. Challenges continue in these countries with respect to intellectual property and contractual rights, as well as regulatory and reimbursement processes. However, many of these items continue to evolve with regulatory reform and cross-border collaborations creating opportunities for medical device innovators from the USA and Europe. These markets promise to be the largest in the world by 2050. Though they each spend considerably less per capital on health care than the USA, meaning per unit pricing may be a challenge to new companies, their collective middle class is forecasted to be twice as large as the G7 countries combined by 2020 [14, 15]. Populations this large with new wealth will need advanced healthcare options and present more space to compete.

Innovation Support

According to the Innovation Learning Network [16], there are over 100 innovation centers in the USA devoted to healthcare with their own membership made up of healthcare systems, health foundations, safety net providers, design/innovation firms, and tech companies. Couple this with the various translational medicine institutes at most academic medical centers as well as other leading providers, and the focus on innovation appears high and growing in new ways. These entities are bringing financial resources from the organizations directly as well as partnerships with investment firms. They also bring facilities, expertise, and access to patients. The new combination of expertise is meant to seek and develop technologies needed by providers and health systems utilizing their input from the outset. Since many medical devices emanate from academic medical centers and many future ones are likely to come from large, multihospital systems, these new models of collaborative financing show promise.

Regulatory Reforms

Earlier reviews of the FDA pointed to two major areas challenging medical device companies: poor interactions and slow processes. In an effort to improve collaborations with developers and field experts, the FDA has instituted a number of pilot projects such as the following, all showing promise in improving relationships between developers and regulators:

- Expedited Access Pathway Program [17]
- FDA-TRACK Program Areas and Dashboards [18]
- Third Party Review [19]
- Medical Device Single Audit Program (MDSAP) Pilot [20]

Possibly more promising are the reforms aimed at improving review and approval times. In "FDA Exempts 120 Medical Device Types from Most Regulation" posted June 30, 2015, Alexander Gaffney, RAC reports the FDA is showing its intent to exempt many devices from pre-market notification requirements as provided in its new final guidance document, "Intent to Exempt Certain Unclassified, Class II, and Class I Reserved Medical Devices from Premarket Notification Requirements" [21]. Though many are low-risk devices, the direction of removing the heavier burden of a 510(k) process for some devices could be an indication of a more flexible agency [22].

In addition, the US House of Representatives approved in May 2015 H.R. 1455 "Speeding Access to Already Approved Pharmaceutics Act" [23]. Though not dealing with devices, the direction is a promising one for taking technologies approved in other areas and reducing US approval times by relying more on the process used elsewhere.

The most sweeping legislation may be H.R. 6 "The 21st Century Cures Act," which is a broad sweeping piece legislation that incorporates items from a number of other bills submitted in the last couple of years [24]. On the drug side, there are items related to reliance on surrogate endpoints and biomarkers that will no doubt raise concerns. In addition, there is a directive to consider other, nontraditional study designs. For medical devices, however, there are a number of sections that hold promise that the FDA is moving in the right direction. Examples include the ability to designate certain devices as "breakthrough" technologies providing them with faster reviews and earlier market entry based on early data and lack of suitable alternatives. There is the possibility of using patient-reported data, including in the postapproval phase, which can change the dynamic and expense of data collection in many cases. To promote innovation, there is a 3 % annual increase to the NIH's budget as well as a newly created "Innovation Fund" allocated $2 Billion a year for 5 years. Though the final approval of H.R.6 has not occurred, it has bilateral support and points in many promising directions.

A final promising, and practical, note on the regulatory side comes with the approval of both the Edwards Lifesciences Sapien 3 Transcatheter Heart Valve on June 17, 2015, some 6 months ahead of expectations, and the Medtronic CoreValve Evolut R on June 23, 2015 [25–27].

Patent Reforms

Another piece of "The 21st Century Cures Act" addresses the addition of patent exclusivity time for certain technologies and devices. These can be of considerable value to a company. However, this is an active legislative area and where turmoil and confusion reign at the moment. No less than 14 bills have been introduced in the past 2 years addressing some aspect of patent reform.

The most practical item to actually pass was H.R. 160 "The Protect Medical Innovation Act" voted on June 19, 2015 and passing by a 2 to 1 margin [28]. This bill repeals the medical device excise tax and addresses one of the more painful issues facing US medical device companies, as discussed.

The best summary of such legislation and the status of each can be found at http://www.raps.org/Regulatory-Focus/News/Databases/2015/06/03/20955/FDA-Legislation-Tracker [29]. With much work and debate left, the results are yet to be seen, but there is at least attention to another area where clarity is needed for innovators to have a chance of plotting a successful course.

New Capital Sources

As future support from traditional venture capital sources remains uncertain, other, nontraditional sources look to participate in medical product innovation, offering services, facilities, knowledge, access to patients, and direct capital. As mentioned, the NIH budget may increase, which leads to increased funding to academic medical centers and the FDA is looking to establish an "innovation fund," both of which present opportunity to medical device developers. Since 1982, the US government has provided support via Small Business Innovation Research and Small Business Technology Transfer (SBIR/STTR) programs, encouraging research focused on commercialization in numerous areas with life sciences included [30]. Jonathan J. Fleming of Oxford Biosciences offers in his article "The Decline of Venture Capital Investment in Early-Stage Life Sciences Poses a Challenge to Continued Innovation" [31], recommendations for policies creating targeted areas of interest for such funding (i.e., oncology, cardiovascular disease, neuroscience, etc.). Large health systems, often the leading consumers of medical devices and increasingly more accountable for the economic impact a device provides, look to participate directly in new product innovation, and they have substantial capital to deploy. There are numerous philanthropic funds that take on more direct roles, akin to that more often seen with a VC firm, such as the Coulter Foundation and Broadview Ventures. Finally, various patient advocacy groups have gone beyond awareness campaigns and put significant funds into facilities, research tools, and direct company investments. The Clinical Research Forum, a consortium of academic health systems, professional societies, and medical product manufacturers, commissioned a paper to summarize such efforts in a white paper, "Partnerships with Patient Advocacy Groups/Voluntary Health Organizations Can Bridge Gaps in Clinical Research." [32]

In summary, the funding of medical device innovation is at a crucial juncture. While there may be worrisome trends with respect to the way funding and development have worked in the past, there are signs pointing to a resurgence of certain elements as well as the emergence of new trends and organizations bringing capital and other resources. Innovators are driven to solve problems and challenges. With new funding sources and parameters in the mix, new innovators have new opportunities. A new product, despite its apparent novelty and promise, is not a successful innovation unless part of that innovation includes the means to successfully bring it into the marketplace. Unless a product is successfully commercialized, it will never make it to the patient's bedside in any meaningful way. This new environment presents the opportunity to innovate not just the devices under development but also the methods by which they are developed and brought into the marketplace.

References

1. www.commerce.gov/medical-device-industry-united-states/
2. www.nvca.org. Funding innovation.
3. The MoneyTree™ Report, PriceWaterhouseCoopers and the National Venture Capital Association, 2015.

4. FDA Impact on US Medical Technology Innovation: A Survey of Over 200 Medical Technology Companies, J. Makower et. al. for Stanford University, MDMA, NVCA, and PricewaterhouseCoopers, LLP.

5. Gillenwater T, Calcoen D, Elias L, et al. Taking the pulse of medical device regulation & innovation. California Healthcare Institute and The Boston Consulting Group; 2014.

6. "Table 11.1 Corporate Income tax rate" at www.stats.OECD.org

7. "The U.S. Has the Highest Corporate Income Tax Rate in the OECD" by K. Pomerleau and A. Lundeen at www.taxfoundation.org

8. 26 USC 4191; Health Care and Education Reconciliation Act of 2010, Section 1405 (Public Law 111–152). http://www.gpo.gov/fdsys/pkg/PLAW-111publ152/pdf/PLAW-111publ152.pdf

9. Internal Revenue Service, Final Rule, Taxable Medical Devices, Dec. 7, 2012, 77 FR 72924. See https://www.federalregister.gov/articles/2012/12/07/2012-29628/taxable-medical-devices

10. Ernst & Young, Pulse of the Industry, Medical Technology Report 2012.

11. "Medical Device Manufacture Profits" Medical Policy Brief, Consumer Protection Union, September 2013.

12. Medical Device Manufacturers Association (MDMA – see www.medicaldevices.org)

13. Advanced Medical Technology Association (AdvaMed – see www.advamed.org)

14. "Pulse of the Industry: Differentiating Differently," Medical Technology Report 2014, Ernst and Young.

15. www.globalsherp.org/bric-countries-brics

16. Innovation Learning Network (ILN – see www.innovationlearningnetwork.org)

17. Expedited Access Pathway Program. http://www.fda.gov/medicaldevices/deviceregulationandguidance/howtomarketyourdevice/ucm441467.htm

18. FDA-TRACK Program Areas and Dashboards. http://www.fda.gov/aboutfda/transparency/track/ucm195008.htm

19. Third Party Review. http://www.fda.gov/medicaldevices/deviceregulationandguidance/howtomarketyourdevice/premarketsubmissions/thirdparyreview/default.htm

20. Medical Device Single Audit Program (MDSAP) Pilot. http://www.fda.gov/medicaldevices/internationalprograms/mdsappilot/default.htm

21. "FDA Exempts 120 Medical Device Types from Most Regulation" Posted June 30, 2015, Alexander Gaffney, RAC.

22. Intent to Exempt Certain Unclassified, Class II, and Class I Reserved Medical Devices from Premarket Notification Requirements. http://www.raps.org/Regulatory-Focus/News/2015/06/30/22812/FDA-Exempts-120-Medical-Device-Types-from-Most-Regulation/#sthash.Usp5j3xH.dpuf

23. H.R. 1455 "Speeding Access to Already Approved Pharmaceutics Act."

24. H.R. 6 "The 21st Century Cures Act."

25. www.fda.gov/NewsEvents/Newsroom/PressAnnouncements/ucm451678.htm

26. www.prnewswire.com/news-releases-edwards-recieves-fda-approval-for-sapien-3-transcatheter-heart-valve300101101.html

27. newsroom.medtronic.com/phoenix.zhtml?c=251324&p=irol-newsArticle&ID=2061818

110   R.S. Stack et al.

28. H.R. 160 "The Protect Medical Innovation Act."
29. http://www.raps.org/Regulatory-Focus/News/Databases/2015/06/03/20955/ FDA-Legislation-Tracker
30. www.sbir.gov
31. Jonathan J. Fleming of Oxford Biosciences offers in his article "The decline of venture capital investment in early-stage life sciences poses a challenge to continued innovation". Health Aff 2015;34(2):271–6.
32. Bond G, et.al. Partnerships with patient advocacy groups/Voluntary health organizations can bridge gaps in clinical research by (12/2011). www.clinicalresearchforum.org

11. Corporate Perspective in Surgical Innovation Ethics: A Literature Review

Myriam J. Curet

This chapter provides a review of the literature regarding the ethical issues surrounding the relationships between medicine and industry, with a specific focus on the surgeon and industry relationship. Much has been written on this issue, with opinions ranging from a desire for complete sequestration to the idea that the development of surgical innovations requires these relationships [1–8]. Surgical innovation (novel devices or techniques) is different from medical (drug) innovation in that there is a gradient of novelty that complicates the classification of an innovation as research or therapy [9, 10]. Surgeons often need to modify their technique to match an individual patient's needs or anatomy or may use an already cleared device in a novel manner [11, 12]. The way an innovation is classified affects the level of oversight and regulation needed, and there are not always clear guidelines for determining this classification, sometimes leaving it up to the individual surgeon to [9–15]. "Surgical innovation happens spontaneously and is frequently repeated after it has been introduced" [13]. Another difference is that surgeon experience affects patient outcomes independently of the device or technique used [16]; unlike a new drug, a new device or technique has a learning curve [13–17]. Surgeons determine who needs the surgery and who performs the operations [18]. Some have argued that these differences lead to a greater vulnerability of the surgical patient and require a higher level of trust between the patient and the surgeon [11, 15]. A surgeon's individual judgment, abilities, and personal integrity play a larger role in patient outcomes, making the issue of surgical ethics an important one [11, 13, 16].

© Springer International Publishing Switzerland 2016
S.C. Stain et al. (eds.), *The SAGES Manual Ethics of Surgical Innovation*, DOI 10.1007/978-3-319-27663-2_11

Many of the improvements in surgical care in the past several decades arose through collaboration between surgeons and industry [2, 6, 13]. There is tremendous value in this collaboration and many goals are mutually aligned [19–21]. Existing relationships between industry and academia have resulted in significant innovations and in the distribution of these innovations so that they have become widely available [2, 3, 6, 8, 21–23]. However, past instances of this relationship unduly influencing medical decisions have created debate over what constitutes appropriate guidelines for these relationships or even whether there should be any interaction between industry and physicians, academia, or hospitals [2, 6, 7, 9]. The argument against this type of partnership stems from the belief that the core values of science and medicine of altruism and the pursuit of truth clash with corporate values based on the pursuit of profit [2, 4, 7, 24–26]. Industry has a fiscal responsibility to its shareholders to create a profit and to create enough income to stay in business, whereas the field of medicine is focused on patient-centered care, evidence-based medicine, and continuing education [1, 2, 4, 26–28]. This dichotomy can create the potential for conflicts of interest (or perceived conflicts of interest) [4, 7, 26]. Critics of industry and physician interactions have a fundamental distrust of the profit motive in medicine [6]. However, it is possible for these seemingly competing interests to balance [2, 6]. In addition, some have argued that industry and academia ultimately share the same value of improved patient care [6, 27]. Companies with a long-term outlook understand that continued growth is dependent on providing a high-quality product that provides a service or fills a need [26]. While it is important to acknowledge that industry is motivated to sell products, a company's enduring success is tied to the quality of patient care provided by using their products and to the professionalism of investigators and surgeons [2, 6]; "the true interest of industry is served only by unbiased research" [27]. Both physicians and industry want effective medications and devices that benefit patients, maximize care (benefits, effectiveness), and minimize harm and legal risks [6, 19]. Industry should partner with physicians and be treated as an equal, and industry and surgeons must have an open and honest dialog with each other [17].

This chapter will review the literature that outlines the history of these relationships, as well as areas of intersection such as product development, research, training/education, dissemination of results from corporate-sponsored research, sales representatives in the operating room, the basis for conflicts, and current guidelines used to manage the potential for conflicts of interest.

History

In the 1950s and 1960s, governmental financial support of research was plentiful and very little funding came from industry [7]. However, attitudes began to shift toward a more favorable view of industry financing in the late 1970s [7]. Laws were passed to encourage this transition, protecting intellectual property rights and allowing universities to patent discoveries resulting from federally funded research (the Bayh-Dole Act of 1980) [7]. In 1993, industry supported 7 % of university research and development in all scientific fields [29]. In 1996, over 90 % of life science companies in the USA had some relationship with academia with nearly 60 % supporting university research and nearly 40 % supporting education of students and fellows [20]. By 2007, industry was funding the majority (58 %) of biomedical research [30], and by 2011, this had increased to 63 % [31]. Industry funding has been especially important for applied research and for development, accounting for 53 % of funding for applied research and 78 % for development in 2011 [31]. This support has been a driving factor in maintaining the United States as a global leader in research. The United States is the largest single R&D-performing country in the world, accounting for ~30 % of the global total in 2011 [31]. Compared to other countries, the USA is an early adopter and rapid diffuser of medical technology and the "world's principal engine driving medical advance" [6]. Surgical innovation continues to be important because there are many diseases that still have suboptimal treatments and outcomes [17]. If industry support were removed, the budget of the National Institute of Health would have to be doubled to compensate for the loss in funding [23]. The support is beneficial to companies as well. "More than 60 % of companies who have invested in academic research have recognized patents, products, and sales as a result" [20]. Based on a survey of industry, Blumenthal found that more than half of companies with research investments depend on faculty member to keep staff current with important research, to provide ideas for new products, and, to a lesser extent, to aid in recruiting new researchers. Interestingly, few companies depend on faculty members to invent products the company will license [20].

Product Development

Continued product development and surgical innovations depend on communication between surgeons and industry [5, 17]. Surgeons and industry have access to complementary resources, and each plays a complementary role [20, 26, 27]. Companies depend on user feedback to develop and refine their products to better fit what doctors and patients need, and surgeons require access to company representatives in order to provide that feedback [6]. Companies use the feedback to develop products that are safe, effective, cost-effective, and practical to use. There must be input from both sides for the design, implementation, and refinement of novel surgical devices [27]. This input is crucial for maximizing benefits while minimizing harm and increasing the effectiveness of new devices to better fit the needs of the patient and the surgeon. Blumenthal did find that typically what industry gains when collaborating with investigators, surgeons, and academic institutions is access to new knowledge, ideas, and talented potential staff members rather than marketable inventions [20].

The process of bringing a new product to market involves the design, manufacture, and testing of a product, as well as obtaining regulatory approval and clearances. Research and development of new products is costly and time-consuming, with many dead ends (products that do not pan out or reach the marketing stage) [6, 12, 23]. Academic centers and individual surgeons generally do not have the resources necessary to generate marketable products based on their research [6, 13] and must form alliances with existing companies, or participate in the creation of start-up companies dedicated to developing a specific product. Industry support can help secure funding for future research and can lead to academic ownership of patents and shares of biotech companies [7]. Since the passage of the Bayh-Dole Act in 1980, there have been more than 8,000 companies created as of 2010 to develop academic research and development [13, 32]. Approximately two-thirds of academic institutions hold equity in "start-up" businesses that sponsor research at their institutions [7].

An important part of this process is continual open communication between industry, institutions, and surgeons throughout the product development process. Interaction between medical industries and medical researcher is essential for successful transfer of innovative medications and technologies into clinical practice [21, 22, 26]. AdvaMed (Advanced Medical Technology Association) which represents companies that "develop, produce, manufacture, and market medical products, technologies and related services" gives guidelines in the Code of Ethics on appropriate consulting agreements and payment of royalties [33]. Ownership of intellectual property should be addressed at the onset, prior to exploration, and a royalty agreement should be arranged only where the health care professional has made or is expected to make a novel, significant, or innovative contribution [33]. The significant contribution should be appropriately documented, and payment should not be dependent on requiring purchase of the resulting development [33]. Concern about intellectual property typically arises in cases where a researcher has developed and/or patented a process or device and has obtained industry funding to further develop or promote that device. Most academic institutions have clear policies and procedures for patenting, and these policies will be considered in any contracts with industry [26]. Ownership of data is another area that should be considered and addressed [26]. Most academic institutions have clear policies and procedures already in place that can be followed.

Research

Universities have vested interests in corporate research efforts as these dollars increase the total research portfolio of a university [26]. In addition, corporate sponsorship of high technology research may be very appealing due to the potential for large future profits [26]. "Industry sponsored research can be academically interesting, scientifically valid and publishable" [27]. It can be mutually beneficial to collaborate as industry does not have the infrastructure necessary to conduct clinical research or the necessary access to patients [26]. Academic centers can provide access to patients and have the infrastructure in place to conduct clinical research, but do not have the resources necessary to fund clinical trials [6, 13, 26]. Results of clinical trials conducted through an academic center may be more likely to be published as data collected at an academic center are generally viewed as less prone to bias and are considered more prestigious [26].

It is often difficult to know at the onset whether an innovative procedure or product will turn out to be beneficial or not [11, 13–15]. There are often little data initially [11, 17] and it is critical to gather all data, even initial data [13, 15]. Knight feels all new procedures should start as clinical trials [17]. It has been suggested that pooling data from multiple surgeons performing a novel procedure would allow for a faster determination of the true risks involved [15]. Wall suggests that the safety of new devices should be monitored by requiring all patients in whom devices have been implanted are tracked in a mandatory product registry until the safety of the device has been ascertained [18]. The creation of registries would allow for the identification of potential issues with novel procedures faster and may be even more effective at detecting rare but serious complications than randomized controlled trials, which are often too small and lack the statistical power to capture these low probability events [9]. Involving surgeons at each step of an industry-sponsored clinical trial, from study design to publication or conference presentations, is important for ensuring the independence of research results so that "sponsorship of research is not sponsorship of results" [27]. If this is done so that the surgeon-author participates in trial design, has access to the data, and controls publication, with transparency and the proper disclosures, "research sponsored by industry can be academically interesting, scientifically valid, and publishable" [27]. The publication of the results of clinical trials in peer-reviewed papers is essential for FDA approval [26], as well as for the dissemination of findings to the surgical community. "Clinical research sponsored by medical industry is best conducted under formalized arrangements with contractual rights of sponsor, PI and institution explicitly defined" [21]. According to Mirza, the sponsor must relinquish control over the data, analysis, and results of the clinical research and over the dissemination of research findings [21]. Both the surgeon and industry are better served with these guidelines, as only data and research that is scientifically rigorous will be published. For the individual researcher, numerous concerns result from industry funding of research, which should be considered and addressed including ownership of intellectual property, confidentiality, rapid disclosure of results, publication, and promotion [26]. Corporate sponsorship often is considered biased and not credible because of the direct linkages with industry. This may lead to a reduction of stature in the research community [26]. Furthermore, some referees may write overly negative and biased reviews merely because of corporate sponsorship [26].

Dissemination of Research Results

Concern over the dissemination of results of industry-sponsored research is based on the perception that companies require researchers to keep results private or to delay publications (such as to allow for patent filings) [13, 26, 34]. This is especially of concern when it is felt that negative findings are being suppressed or when it is felt that the company is controlling what is published without disclosure [7, 26, 35].

However, studies have shown that this is not a widespread problem. Companies do not often require researchers to keep results private or to delay publication [34]. In addition, physicians without industry ties also sometimes delay publication of findings or suppress negative results [34]. Delaying publication to protect intellectual property is considered acceptable and is the most common reason cited [34].

Promotion and Advertising

Promotional materials are an integral part of getting any product to the market [6]. This includes product brochures, advertisements, and sales materials, but it also includes research publications. While companies expect that marketing dollars will increase sales, this process need not be contrary to high-quality, evidence-based medicine [6]. In fact, in order to profit long term, it is in the company's best interest to support evidence-based marketing. Promotion and marketing are protected under the US constitution First amendment: freedom of speech which gives companies the right to market and advertise [6]. The Freedom of assembly gives physicians and industry representatives the right to meet and to have mutually beneficial contractual relationships [6]. The Copyright and Patent Clause of the First Amendment protects the rights of companies to enjoy profits that come to their discoveries under patent protection [6]. However, many people are uncomfortable with the idea of profit in health care and see promotion and advertising as antithetical to evidence-based literature [6].

Health Care Industry Representatives

With surgical devices, it is common to have company sales representatives in the operating room to facilitate the safe and efficient use of the device [36]. "Health Care Industry Representatives (HCIR) by virtue of their training, knowledge and expertise can provide technical assistance to the surgical team, which expedites the procedure and facilitates the safe and effective application of surgical products and technologies" [37]. The ACS Statement of Health Care Industry Representatives in the Operating Room supplies guidelines for health care facilities and health care providers to ensure "an optimal surgical outcome, as well as the patient's safety, right to privacy, and confidentiality when a HCIR is present during a surgical procedure" [37]. The Statement gives guidance on facility requirements, as well as roles and limitations of the HCIR in the operating room. The statement explicitly mentions that HCIRs should be informed as to expected behavior in the operating room, should be informed of and meet the facilities' requirements for being in the OR and should refrain from giving surgical or medical advice. Some authors have suggested the additional safeguard of informing the patient and gaining their consent prior to allowing industry representatives in the operating room during the surgical procedure [36, 37].

Sudarsky states that concerns have been raised about the influence of HCIR visits on physicians [5]. Increased visits can lead to increased use of a company's product. HCIRs tend to present positive information about product and may omit unfavorable information. Johnson and Rogers state that there is evidence that surgeons are more tolerant of conflicts of interest than medical physicians and feels this is due to the fact that industry representatives are frequently part of the theater team, regarded as colleagues and friends [35].

Training and Education

"Companies have a responsibility to make training and education of their products and Medical Technologies available to Health Care Professionals" [33]. "In fact, the US food and Drug Administration mandates training and education to facilitate the safe and effective use of certain Medical Technologies" [33]. AdvaMed Code of Ethics has principles which help guide companies when conducting training and education programs on medical technologies for health care professionals [33].

Industry has a vested interest in the quality of education of the next generation of physicians, so educational programs specifically designed for residents and fellows may be an area of investment for companies [27]. A 2007 national survey of department chairs found that 37 % of clinical departments received residency or fellowship training support from industry [38]. In some disciplines, industry funding has increased the number of residency spots available, which can alleviate doctor shortages [13, 25]. For example, the dermatology residency program at Stanford University accepted industry money as a way to fund an increased number of residency slots [25]. Concerns were raised about whether this industry support would unduly influence residents. Companies are trying to increase the market for their products, and critics remain skeptical about the altruism of industry in this situation [25].

Much attention has been paid to industry influence on Continuing Medical Education (CME). In 2006, 67 % of CME was covered by commercial support, equaling about 1.2 billion dollars, which was 4 times the amount it was in 1998 [13, 28]. To ensure that educational materials are evidenced-based and are not biased, current CME accreditation guidelines do not allow for industry suggestion of speakers or overview/influence on content [1]. There are also now guidelines restricting activity to educational activities that are carefully segregated in space and time in contact with industry representatives [6, 13, 19, 39, 40]. Both the Council of Medical Specialty Societies and the ACS have developed guidelines for industry and society collaborations for support of CME that clearly state the need for educational content to be independent of industry influence [19, 39]. Both statements give guidelines on various aspects of industry support in CME programs [19, 39]. In addition, AdvaMed and PhRMA (Pharmaceutical Research and Manufacturers of America) also address appropriate interactions between industry representatives and CME sponsors in their Codes of Ethics [33, 41].

"The 2004 ACCME Standards for Commercial Support: Standards to Ensure Independence in CME Activities (Accreditation Criteria 7–10) are designed to ensure that CME activities are independent and free of commercial bias. The Standards impose stringent restrictions on CME providers' interactions with drug/device companies and other companies the ACCME defines as a commercial interest. The ACCME allows providers to accept company funding for CME activities, but prohibits any commercial influence, direct or indirect, over CME content. Building on guidelines that the ACCME first issued in 1987 and formally adopted in 1992, the 2004 ACCME Standards for Commercial Support comprise six Standards: Independence, Resolution of Personal Conflicts of Interest, Appropriate Use of Commercial Support, Appropriate Management of Associated Commercial Promotion, Content and Format without Commercial Bias, and Disclosures Relevant to Potential Commercial Bias" [40].

When making decisions about implementing the ACCME Standards for Commercial Support, the ACCME says that CME providers must always defer to independence from commercial interests, transparency, and the separation of CME from product promotion. In other words, the purpose of CME must be to serve physicians' learning and practice needs and to promote public health [40]. Both the AdvaMed and PhRMA codes emphasize these same points, saying that educational grants should be paid only to organizations with a "genuine educational function," companies should reimburse only legitimate educational activities, that the conference sponsor should "independently control and be responsible for the selection of program content, faculty, educational methods and materials," that only modest meals and expenses should be reimbursed, that noneducational branded promotional items or gifts should not be given, and that funding should not be offered to compensate for the time spent by health care professionals in the CME event [33, 41].

Paying for a physician's travel expenses to education symposium used to be very common, but in response to public outcry over lavish and clearly inappropriate gifts from industry to surgeons, strict guidelines prohibiting any type or size gift or reimbursement of any kind were suggested and implemented [1, 22]. There may be instances where physician reimbursement by industry is appropriate such as when a surgeon is learning a new surgical technique [22, 33, 35, 41], and in some cases, guidelines have been revised to recognize these instances. However, reimbursement should be limited to necessary expenses that are able to withstand public scrutiny and must not require or imply that the surgeon must then use that technology [1, 22, 33, 35, 41].

Conflicts of Interest

The reason for concern over industry relationships with the medical community stems from the idea of undue influence and that these relationships can create conflicts of interest [2, 13, 21]. A surgeon or university with financial interest in a company or in the success of a surgical device has two interests: the interests of the patient and their own financial interests [1, 7, 28]. Sometimes these interests will be complementary and will align, such as when a new treatment is clearly an improvement over the standard of care. It is when these interests conflict that there is concern that they may impact decision-making in a way to cause patient harm [35]. Conflicts of interest can be real or perceived and can exist between surgeons and industry, between hospitals and industry, or between surgeons and patients [26]. They can be a problem when they influence choice of treatment, such as when the needs of the patient are not put above all others, or by affecting the accuracy of an assessment of risk (i.e., patient informed choice) [28]. Ideally, in cases where these interests are at odds with each other, the needs of the patient will outweigh corporate and surgeon self-interests [22, 26].

The problem is rarely with intentional bias, where a surgeon knowingly chooses a medical procedure or device solely due to their financial ties with the company, which would be, "unprofessional, unethical, and potentially fraudulent" [1, 4, 7, 21, 42].

However, unconscious or unintentional preferences based on financial and nonfinancial factors can still influence decision-making [1, 28]. For example, a surgeon might choose a particular medical device because they feel an unconscious need to return the favor after receiving gifts or consulting or speaker fees (the principle of reciprocity) [1, 2, 4, 7, 13, 35]. This is especially an issue when the gift or payment is lavish or extreme [1, 22], but occurs even with small gifts [2]. Well-meaning professionals can find it hard to resist the unconscious influence of incentives [42]. Scientists funded by industry produce studies which are more favorable to new products than those whose funding is independent of industry [7, 8]. Surgeons with a financial interest in a company are more likely to report on off-label use of devices and products [5].

There have been cases that were morally suspect and these have eroded public trust [4]. A history of vacation trips, concerts, and large royalty or consultant fees from industry to physicians [13] have created a "fundamental distrust of the profit motive in medicine, with any benefit that comes to physicians through industry contact being suspect" [6]. A gift of any kind forms a relationship, making the recipient indebted to the giver. The strength of this debt varies, but at some level it becomes a bribe when an over generous gift is given with "strings attached" [2].

However, this feeling of a need for reciprocity can be lessened when the financial amount is appropriate and has been earned or is a reimbursement of actual and reasonable expenses. It is then no longer a gift or favor, but is then the return on investment of time, expertise, etc. [21, 22, 35]. When a surgeon develops a new device, they should be compensated [21–23]. IP is the most valued capital in current markets, and innovators are entitled to reap reward for successful results of their creativity and hard work [21]. For other basic science research, financial relationships among sponsor, inventors, and investigators no more compromise the validity of the work than the nonfinancial intrinsic rewards of academic work [21]. Some conflicts are still troublesome, such as when a surgeon involved in creating a new product is compensated with equity in a start-up company making that device and is the same surgeon conducting the clinical trials for that device [22]. Oversight to confirm that the compensation is appropriate can help prevent some of these conflicts [3, 35].

There are also nonfinancial factors in play. Surgeons may feel pressured to innovate, from a personal desire to succeed, patient demand, competition with colleagues, insurance payers, or from their academic institution [11, 13]. This can cause internal conflicts of interest created by the surgeon that are not the result of direct industry involvement.

These nonfinancial factors can include a surgeon's emotional satisfaction and excitement from making a new discovery and advancing the science of medicine, or enhanced reputation and academic advancement from the dissemination and publication of new information [1, 14, 15, 17, 28, 35]. Academic institutions also need public recognition to gain funding (from governmental and private donors, as well as from industry) and may push surgeons to innovate in an attempt to become recognized as a "center of excellence" [7, 13]. Conflicts do not involve just surgeons and industry, but academic centers can also be conflicted [7, 8, 28]. Schafer gives examples of prestigious universities who have made millions from their ownership of shares in companies with which they have commercial agreements [7]. The President of Johns Hopkins University stated that "to move your research forward, you've got to do partnerships with industry" [7] and the former vice dean of research stated that Hopkins has become "one of the biggest biotech companies in the world" [7].

It is also human nature to give preference to those with whom we have a positive relationship, even when no money has exchanged hands [4, 28]. As mentioned previously, it has been suggested that the practice of allowing company sales representatives in the operating room (a practice common for device manufacturers more than for pharmaceutical companies) creates a favorable relationship between the surgeon and the company representative that can effect decision-making [35].

Publications detailing company malfeasance exist including fraudulent and illegal activities [4, 13, 22, 35]. Money spent by industry on promotion and advertising has increased, and some references have stated that twice as much money is spent on promotion than on research and development [2, 22, 28, 43]. Hockenberry used data from Department of Justice lawsuit to describe the extent of orthopedic surgeon's financial relationships with implant manufacturers [3]. Hockenberry found that the number of orthopedic surgeons receiving payments declined substantially with an increase in proportion of surgeons who had academic affiliation, but still the payments represented 25 % of an average orthopedic surgeon's annual income. He concluded that concern seemed warranted although payments went to only 4 % of practicing orthopedic surgeons [3]. The Department of Justice settlement required each company to have an onsite federal monitor, systematically evaluate their consulting arrangements, ensure that consulting physicians publically disclosed their financial engagement to patients, and publicly disclose the name, location, and amount of money paid to each surgeon or organization on their respective web sites [3]. Lichter says that companies are looking for access, influence, and gratitude and data show that this spending does have an influence on surgeons, physicians, academic institutions, and even societies [28].

Managing Conflict

Disclosure is key to managing conflict [2, 11, 13, 21, 23, 26, 35, 42]. In fact, disclosure of principal investigators' financial ties to industry is required by FDA [8, 23, 27]. Disclosure as a first step can lead to the identification of payments for services that are ethically suspect, such as payment for simply using a product, and can lead to the creation of policies limiting interactions to those deemed appropriate. Disclosure is essential: [35] by creating transparency, it becomes possible to question the relationships, payments, or interactions and to then choose those that are considered reasonable and manageable and to put policies in place that prevent or prohibit those that are deemed inappropriate. There also needs to be systems in place to confirm compliance; currently, disclosure requires self-reporting [22, 26, 35]. There is a need for a policy to manage justifiable interactions and prohibit those that cannot be justified [35]. Some have argued that disclosure alone is not enough, and that it provides a false sense that the conflict has been adequately dealt with [11], when in fact, it may do, "nothing to remedy or mitigate their potentially biasing effects" [35, 44]. In addition, the disclosure of a conflict of interest, "shifts the burden onto the recipient of the information" [35], such as the reader of a journal article, or a patient, who may not be able to fully understand or to process the significance or possible consequences of the stated/disclosed conflict of interest [1]. Raad states that there is little evidence that disclosure requirements are meaningful to the recipients of the information [8]. Loewenstein expresses concern about reliance on disclosure as a means to manage conflict [42]. He states that "disclosure has appeal... because it acknowledges the problem of conflicts but involves minimal regulation and is less expensive to implement than more comprehensive remedies" [42]. He states that when disclosure occurs, patients may take the disclosed fact of their physicians have been paid by ...companies as an indication that those physicians must be experts" [42]. Patients may believe that physicians are biased by conflicts but not their physician. Disclosure can also increase the pressure on patients to go along with the advice, thus decreasing the trust in the clinician's advice but increasing the pressure to take the advice so as not to make physician feel the patient distrusts him [42]. He goes on to suggest that to make disclosure more effective, certain efforts should be made, such as obtaining unconflicted second opinions, providing disclosure by third parties, giving the patient time to reflect on the advice, and letting the patient make the decision while not in the presence of the physician [42].

Policies have now been put in place by universities and journal editors to require research independence and full disclosure [7, 26, 42]. For example, the International Committee of Medical Journal Editors requests that authors disclose all financial ties, participate in trial design, have access to data, and control publication [1, 7, 8]. To further address these concerns, increasing transparency when industry is involved with publication is also necessary, including identifying company writers, making industry personnel authors on publications [26] and submitting articles to peer-reviewed journals as original research with all conflicts of interest stated.

Additional measures have been proposed such as insulating certain aspects of medical or research decision-making from industry influence such as has been done with CME [8]. Raad has also proposed independent oversight of academic work, making sure that no one company has excessive say, limiting the time that faculty can send on outside activities and limiting the monetary value of payments that academics may receive from their relationship with industry. Over three-quarters of medical schools use these strategies [8].

Guidelines, Regulations, and Oversight

Rigorous regulation of surgical innovation and independent ethic review and oversight is resisted by surgeons, institution, some surgical associations, and industry [11]. Multiple societies and organizations have developed guidelines [2–4, 12, 13, 21, 42], including American Medical Association, Medical Advisory commission, American College of Surgeons, American College of Emergency Physicians, American Academy of Orthopedic Surgeons, and the Society of University Surgeons. Industry societies such as Pharmaceutical Research and Manufacturers of America and AdvaMed have also developed guidelines or Code of Ethics [33, 41]. Companies who are members of AdvaMed "are strongly encouraged to follow the seven elements of an effective compliance program, appropriately tailored for each Company, namely: (1) implementing written policies and procedures; (2) designating a compliance officer and compliance committee; (3) conducting effective training and education; (4) developing effective lines of communication (including an anonymous reporting function); (5) conducting internal monitoring and auditing; (6) enforcing standards through well-publicized disciplinary guidelines; and (7) responding promptly to detected problems and undertaking corrective action" [31]. Due to all of the above-mentioned concerns, many universities have policies in place for disclosure of conflicts of interest, for public accounting of all commercial support to a facility, and for limits on commercial holdings by researchers [28]. In addition, disclosure of financial ties is now routinely expected as part of an introduction during conference presentations. Laws have also been passed to regulate conflicts of interest, such as the Sunshine Act, which requires drug and device manufacturers to publically disclose any compensation to physicians or teaching hospitals that is over $10 [13, 43, 44].

There is wide discretion in how all of these guidelines are interpreted [28]. "Notably, the AMA conducted a campaign to educate physicians about its guidelines (on industry) interactions and much of the campaign was funded by pharmaceutical companies" [22, 28].

With all of this public disclosure, are conflicts of interest still an issue? Some have argued that a third party should regulate HC-industry relationship. This was done in Massachusetts and had a negative impact on the economy, so the code of conduct was changed to allow more interaction [5]. The question becomes, is self-policing sufficient or are governmental regulations necessary? [11] The answer comes from the level to which companies are successful at self-regulating [45]. Systems that have shown success are those where, "top management commits to an ethics program," which has the effect of establishing, "formal control systems that standardize the behavior of employees within an organization and facilitate compliance with ethics codes and standards" [45]. Governmental regulations do not apply to all research, such as that which is privately funded or surgical innovations that are considered part of the routine, therapeutic practice of surgery. Classifying all surgical innovations as experimental (requiring research oversight) can be problematic in that it may prevent insurance reimbursement, which could ultimately harm the patient [9]. Therefore, self-regulation by the surgeon and by industry in some form will always be necessary.

Regulations and guidelines designed to balance the interests of industry with those of the public are useful and facilitate the surgeon-industry relationship; however, regulations designed to force companies to act in an altruistic manner are unrealistic. More realistic is the ideal of excellent service: putting the customers' interests first, integrity to the company's mission and values, and honest and ethical business practices [6].

Conclusion

This chapter provides a review of the literature regarding the ethical issues surrounding the relationships between medicine and industry, with a specific focus on the surgeon and industry relationship. The relationship is complex. Industry and the medical profession must work together to increase scientific rigor, integrity, and transparency with the goal of improving health care through expanded access to information and unbiased research.

References

1. Foster RS. Conflict of interest: recognition, disclosure and management. J Am Coll Surg. 2003;196:505–17.
2. Iserson KV, Cerfolio RJ, Sade RM. Politely refuse the pen and note pad: gifts from industry to physicians harm patients. Ann Thor Surg. 2007;84:1077–84.
3. Hockenberry JM, Weigel P, Auerbach A, et al. Financial payments by orthopedic device makers to orthopedic surgeons. Arch Intern Med. 2011;171:1759–65.
4. Marco CA, Moskop JC, Solomon RC, et al. Gifts to physicians from pharmaceutical industry: an ethical analysis. Ann Emerg Med. 2006;48:513–21.
5. Sudarsky D, Charania J, Inman A, et al. The impact of industry representative's visits on utilization of coronary stents. Am Heart J. 2013;166:258–65.
6. Nakayama DK. In defense of industry-physician relationships. Am Surg. 2010;76:987–94.
7. Schafer A. Biomedical conflicts of interest: a defence of the sequestration thesis-learning from the cases of Nancy Olivieri and David Healy. J Med Ethics. 2004;30:8–24.
8. Raad R, Appelbaum PS. Relationships between medicine and industry: approaches to the problem of conflicts of interest. Annu Rev Med. 2012;65:465–77.
9. Mastroianni AC. Liability, regulation and policy in surgical innovation: the cutting edge of research and therapy. Health Matrix Clevel. 2006;16:351–442.
10. Rogers WA, Lotz M, Hutchison K, et al. Identifying surgical innovation: a qualitative study of surgeons' view. Ann Surg. 2014;259:273–8.
11. Dixon JB, Logue J, Komesaroff PA. Promises and ethical pitfalls of surgical innovation: the case of bariatric surgery. Obes Surg. 2013;23:1698–702.

12. Biffl WL, Spain DA, Reitsma AM, et al. Responsible development and application of surgical innovations: a position statement of the Society of University Surgeons. J Am Coll Surg. 2008;206:1204–9.

13. Lee WT, Rocke D, Holsinger FC. Surgical innovation, industry partnership, and the enemy within. Head Neck. 2014;36:461–5.

14. Morreim H, Mack MJ, Sade RM. Surgical innovation: too risky to remain unregulated? Ann Thorac Surg. 2006;82:1957–65.

15. Angelos P. Surgical ethics and the challenge of surgical innovation. Am J Surg. 2014;208:881–5.

16. Ergina PL, Cook JA, Blazeby JM, et al. Challenges in evaluating surgical innovation. Lancet. 2009;374(9695):1097–104.

17. Knight JL. Ethics: the dark side of surgical innovation. Innovations (Phila). 2012;7:307–13.

18. Wall LL, Brown D. The perils of commercially driven surgical innovation. Am J Obstet Gynecol. 2010;202:30.e1–4

19. Statement on Guidelines for Collaboration of Industry and Surgical Organizations in Support of Continuing Education. www.facs.org/about-acs/statements/36-collaboration-industry-surgical

20. Blumenthal D, Causino N, Campbell E, et al. Relationships between academic institutions and industry in the life sciences – an industry survey. N Engl J Med. 1996;334:368–73.

21. Mirza SK. Accountability of the accused: facing public perceptions about financial conflicts of interest in spine surgery. Spine J. 2004;4:491–4.

22. Epps, CH, Jr. Ethical guidelines for orthopaedists and industry. Clin Orthop Relat Res. 2003;(412):14–20.

23. Lieberman I, Herndon J, Hahn J, et al. Surgical innovation and ethical dilemmas: a panel discussion. Cleve Clin J Med. 2008;75 Suppl 6:S13–21.

24. Lewis S, Baird P, Evans RG, et al. Dancing with the porcupine: rules for governing the university-industry relationship. CMAJ. 2001;165:783–5.

25. Kuehn, BM. Pharmaceutical industry funding for residencies sparks controversy. JAMA. 2005; 293:1572–80. Brand RA, Buckwalter JA, Talman CL, et al. Industrial support of orthopaedic research in the academic setting. Clin Orthop Relat Res. 2003:45–53.

26. Brand RA, Buckwalter JA, Talman CL, et al. Industrial support of orthopaedic research in the academic setting. Clin Ortho Relat Res. 2003;412:45–53.

27. Crowninshield, R. The orthopaedic profession and industry: conflict or convergence of interests. Clin Orthop Relat Res. 2003;(457):8–13.

28. Lichter PR. Debunking myths in physician-industry conflicts of interest. Am J Ophthalmol. 2008;146:159–71.

29. National Science Board. Science & engineering indicators – 1993. Washington, DC: Government Printing Office. 1993. (NSB 93–1).

30. Dorsey ER, de Roulet J, Thompson JP, et al. Funding of US biomedical research, 2003–2008. JAMA. 2010;303:137–43.

31. National Science Board. Science & engineering indicators – 2014. Arlington: National Science Foundation; 2014. (NSB 14–01).

32. Schacht, WH. The Bayh-Dole Act: selected issues in patent policy and the commercialization of technology. 2012.

33. http://advamed.org/res.download/112

34. Blumenthal D, Campbell EG, Anderson MS, et al. Withholding research results in academic life science. Evidence from a national survey of faculty. JAMA. 1997;277:1224–8.

35. Johnson J, Rogers W. Joint issues--conflicts of interest, the ASR hip and suggestions for managing surgical conflicts of interest. BMC Med Ethics. 2014;15:63.

36. Sillender M. Can patients be sure they are fully informed when representatives of surgical equipment manufacturers attend their operations? J Med Ethics. 2006;32:395–7.

37. Statement on Health Care Industry Representatives in the Operating Room. https://facs.org/about-acs-statements-33-industry-reps-in-or Code

38. Campbell EG, Weissman JS, Ehringhaus S, et al. Institutional academic industry relationships. JAMA. 2007;298:1779–86.

39. Council of Medical Specialty Societies Code for Interactions with Companies. http://www.cmss.org/codeforinteractions.aspx

40. http://www.accme.org/requirements/accreditation-requirements-cme-providers/standards-for-commercial-support

41. http://www.phrma.org/sites/default/files/pdf/phrma_marketing_code_2008.pdf

42. Loewenstein G, Sah S, Cain DM. The unintended consequences of conflict of interest disclosure. JAMA. 2012;307:669–70.

43. American Medical Association. Sunshine Act frequently asked questions. Available from: http://www.ama-assn.org/ama/pub/advocacy/topics/sunshine-act-and-physician-financial-transparency-reports/sunshine-act-faqs.page. Accessed 16 Apr 2015.

44. Lipworth W, Kerridge I, Morrell B, et al. Views of health journalists, industry employees and news consumers about disclosure and regulation of industry-journalist relationships: an empirical ethical study. J Med Ethics. 2015;41:252–7.

45. Arnold DG, Oakley JL. The politics and strategy of industry self-regulation: the pharmaceutical industry's principles for ethical direct-to-consumer advertising as a deceptive blocking strategy. J Health Polit Policy Law. 2013;38:505–44.

12. Innovations in Surgery: Responsibilities and Ethical Considerations

Lee L. Swanström

There are many facets to surgical innovation—not least of which is the personality of surgeons who actively practice innovation. On one level, surgery is defined by innovation. One of the elements in surgery that makes it an art as opposed to a rote technical practice is the fact that surgeons continuously change and adapt their practice. During a case, if a surgeon encounters nontextbook anatomy or a novel problem, they are required to *innovate* their way around the problem. Likewise, we have a practice and a culture that makes us continuously review what and how we do things. It is the rare surgeon who, after years in practice, still performs his operations the way he did at the start of his practice. The changes made during the evolution of one's techniques are iterative innovations based on his cumulative experience, outcomes (good and bad), and new technologies that happen along. This continuous evolution of techniques based on the infinite clinical variety of the human milieu is, in fact, what makes it almost impossible to create high-fidelity virtual reality simulators that seem remotely realistic or useful to surgeons and so frustrates the software engineers developing them. There are a few `and, in fact, the surgeon who did not evolve his techniques or was unable to innovate around intraoperative "surprises" would be a poor surgeon and while not "unethical" certainly fails in his responsibilities to his patients.

A more interesting situation exists when a surgeon has the opportunity, the inclination, or the ambition to introduce truly disruptive innovations into practice. All human *métiers* (callings? professions?) have their pioneers, an *avant garde*, but they differ according to their focus—which in turn is probably based on their degree of social responsibility, measured by their potential physical threat to their fellow citizens. I often use as an example—just to lend contrast to the discussion of the *avant garde*—of the fine arts. With few exceptions, art seldom presents a physical threat to the public—it may incite social turmoil with subsequent physical consequence, but this is quite remote from the individual act of creating "art." While the craftsmanship of fine arts is always admired and is what is after all taught, what is truly valued in art is the innovative. There are three "outcome measures" in the art world: success in one's own time, whether one is remembered after one's own time, and current marketability. Most people today are familiar with the big names in art: Praxiteles of Athens, Leonardo da Vinci, Caravaggio, Rembrandt, Monet, Van Gogh, even to Warhol and Damien Hirst. Why is this? Why does their art sell for millions while the thousands or tens of thousands of their contemporaries are totally forgotten? By and large, it is because they were innovators. They are identified with a turning point in the progress of the art that had a lasting significance. They also tend to be troubled or trouble makers as well, and such notoriety seldom hurts the fine artist. As we have already mentioned though, as fine arts present no tangible threat, by and large, to those who interact with the artist, this opens the door for a generalized drive for artists to be identified as the innovator and leads to the cultural norm in the world of fine arts for the artist to be a "rebel" or "outrageous"—the superficial trappings of the true pivotal innovator.

Surgery, on the other hand, because of its responsibility for individual patient's lives or well-being, is, by and large, a conservative field. The steady-state for surgeons is to practice as they were taught and to have very rigid protocols for altering how they do things: Evidence-based guidelines and a general respect for tradition are cultural norms for the world of surgery. None the less, we as a profession are attracted to the idea of "new" or "innovative" and often seek out education opportunities or meetings specifically to hear and see the latest procedures or technologies. In addition, we are all familiar with innovative surgeons, and they are often something of "rockstars" in the surgery world (Fig. 12.1). Thus, there are inherent tensions in the world of surgery—tradition and a moral imperative to change slowly what we do, a need to innovate constantly to keep up with technology and "innovate around immediate problems", natural human resistance to having to change

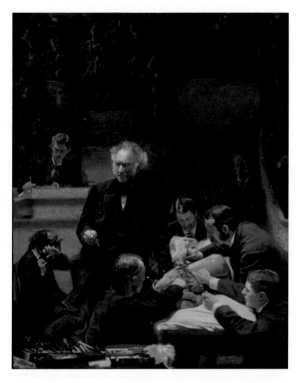

Fig. 12.1. Painting of an early famous surgeon "rockstar." (Thomas Eakins, Portrait of Dr. Samuel D. Gross [The Gross Clinic] Google Art Project." Licensed under Public Domain via Commons – https://commons.wikimedia.org/ wiki/File:Thomas_Eakins,_American_-_Portrait_of_Dr._Samuel_D._Gross_ (The_Gross_Clinic)_-_Google_Art_Project.jpg#/media/File:Thomas_Eakins,_ American_-_Portrait_of_Dr._Samuel_D._Gross_(The_Gross_Clinic)_-_ Google_Art_Project.jpg).

routine vs the sexiness of surgical pioneers. Overall though, the vast majority of surgeons change their practice slowly and carefully, and only dream of being a surgical pioneer or rockstar....

So what of those surgical pioneers, those who report on the first of something, those who take time from practice to develop a new technology or procedure, or travel to far places to see the new and then bring it home and then simply start doing it. As we all know someone like this, it is pretty easy to create a general profile of such a surgeon: bright, questioning, driven, often personally eccentric, typically a "serial pioneer," frequently admired and sought after to headline meetings and very often, in trouble in his local situation. Sociologists have shown that the incidence of true innovators (or "geniuses") across all professions is more or less equal and accounts for between 1 and 4 % of the practitioners in the field [1]. However, there is also recognition that some of the defining traits of the innovative personality can come close to DSM-5 pathologic conditions diagnosis of narcissism, personality disorder, etc.

The source therefore of the friction with the innovator's local environment seems to be that the drive or compulsion to innovate is such a priority it can, at times, supersede the impulses to maintain a social order or even—in the worst of cases—the sacred responsibility that we hold to the patient. This can lead to abrasive interactions within the health system, financial self-harm, and, again in the worst cases, harm to an individual patient. Even in the event of no harm to the patient, or even luckily demonstrable success in bettering patient care, innovators are typically greeted with ill acceptance or even violent denigration. This phenomenon is also well described by sociologists. In this regard, there exists both the occasional focus on the more maladaptive aspects of the innovator (stubbornness, obsessiveness, lack of regard for others, etc) and the well-described social reaction to innovative change. At times, the sociologic portrait of the innovator can approach viciousness as evidenced by the following quote: "First, research suggests that true innovators (the first 2–3 % adopters) are more likely to be social deviants, abnormal in their epistemic drive, and adopt innovations indiscriminately rather than based on any rational choice calculus. Why should we understand and emulate their behavior?" [2] The second and well-researched phenomenon is society's natural resistance to change. E. M. Rogers first defined this in 1962 with his famous "adoption bell-curve" showing classic social resistance to the new [3].

This was recently expressed in surgical terms by Thomas Krummel [4], who defined the general reactions to surgical innovation as follows:

- Abject Horror—"Are you out of your mind!?"
- Swift Denunciation—"It's not just a bad idea—it's Dangerous"
- Begrudging Acceptance—"There may be limited Applications…"
- Ringing Endorsement—"I actually Proposed this 10 years ago" (Fig. 12.2)

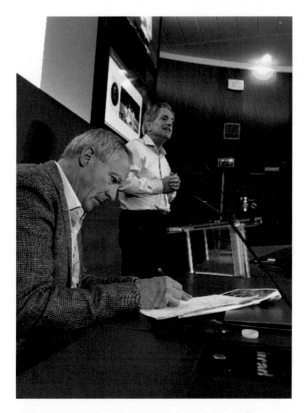

Fig. 12.2. Tom Krummel (*left*) at the 2015 BEST Innovation Symposium, Strasbourg, France. (Courtesy of the author).

Case Study

A perfect illustration of the difficulties faced by the surgical innovator is the contemporaneous example of the surgeon Erich Mühe. Erich Mühe (born 1938) is widely accepted as the first to perform laparoscopic cholecystectomy in 1985. From the beginning, he was innovative and inquisitive and fit the innovator/surgeon profile as he produced multiple medical innovations during training at Erlangen University. Most notably, prior to laparoscopic cholecystectomy, he was the design of a "bed-cycle" to prevent postoperative DVT [5]. In fact, as a passionate bicyclist he created several innovations to bicycling. From the beginning he had problems. His inquisitiveness eventually marginalized him from

Erlangen—a small but prestigious university program—and he ended up at Böblingen hospital—a small community institution. His position there was rather isolated, but he continued to invent—eventually designing the "galloscope" system to perform laparoscopic and later gasless laparoscopic surgery. His remarkable accomplishments were initially ignored by the German surgical establishment. His attempts to publish his experience were uniformly rejected, and the few presentations he was allowed were brutally criticized. After nearly 100 cases, he had a patient who died of complications and this opened the door for professional criticism—which arrived quickly and virulently [6]. A costly law suit, loss of referrals, and continued criticism by establishment surgeons led to destruction of his practice, marital difficulties, and essentially, by his description while relating this history during the Storz lecture at SAGES in 1999, ruined his career. Ironically enough, he much later received commendation by the German Surgical Society. He died relatively young in 2005, fairly disillusioned and somewhat bitter.

Overall, one is left with the perhaps unanswerable question of whether the surgeon/innovator is a sociopath, a "rockstar," a victim, or something of all three.

Patient's Perspective

From the standpoint of the patient, surgical innovation represents both an opportunity and a risk. Many patients naturally seek out the "latest" and therefore "best" treatments when faced with a chronic or life-threatening problem. "The latest" surgical treatment or technology is naturally expected to be better—either more effective or less invasive, by both the surgeon innovator and by most patients. Obviously this is not always the case. New ideas may turn out to be bad ideas in the long run, and in the short-term, the new in surgery is often associated with a learning curve that not infrequently involves increased complications. From a personal viewpoint on this issue, I had developed a herniated cervical disc as a chief resident, and fresh off of a neurosurgery rotation I was very leery of a standard cervical discectomy and fusion. A somewhat eccentric neurosurgeon in our program had just started performing a less invasive anterior approach, with an annular window and transdiscal hernia reduction, with no fusion. I signed up immediately—even though the procedure had no track record, the surgeon was definitely in his learning curve, and I was immediately acquainted with all the bad things that not infrequently happen with spine surgery. This was partly in desperation from the misery of nerve compression but also from an instinctive desire for something less invasive and newer. Fortunately it turned out well for me, but the procedure itself was later abandoned due to frequent failures and recurrences. Considering the strong psychologic appeal of new procedures to the patient, and the sometimes "driven" desires of the innovator, it is easy to see how ethical proprieties might be bent or broken in the face of the new. Today, there are layers of protection for the patient that often seem meddlesome, burdensome, and obstructive to the innovator—and which probably sometimes are—but that also act as a critical "brake" to an introduction process that in the past was subject to at least overenthusiastic application. There are, on the other hand, external barriers to innovation that, in the name of "patient safety," block innovation purely for self-serving economic reasons. In the United States, the most glaring example of this is the private third party insurance industry, which uses the label of "innovation" or "new" to deny patient coverages purely for economic gain—truly an ethical infraction on a society-wide scale.

Conclusions

Innovation in surgery is a sexy and appealing but potentially hazardous endeavor, both for the patient and the innovative surgeon. The surgical innovator is a flawed, fragile but critical element in the evolution of patient care. Patients are currently fairly well protected from innovative excess by externally imposed processes. The societally imposed ethical protections for patients may be considered burdensome to both the anxious patient and the impetuous innovative surgeon, but probably serve as a useful tool to keep everyone "safe." Constraints on access to the "new" that are imposed or occur as a result of economic interests are certainly unethical and should be condemned. The surgeon innovator on the other hand needs to be recognized for their vital contributions, but we also need to recognize that the drive to innovation can harm the innovator and their patients and, as colleagues, partners, and friends, we need to provide council and support to these creative individuals.

References

1. Kwang R. A big-five personality profile of the adaptor and innovator. J Creat Behav. 2002;36(4):254–68.
2. Sheth JN. The psychology of innovation resistance. Res Mark. 1981;4:273–82.
3. Rogers EM. Diffusion of innovations. 5th ed. New York: Free Press; 2003.
4. IRCAD, Innovations Day, Sept 1, 2015.
5. Reynolds W. The first laparoscopic cholecystectomy. JSLS. 2001;5(1):89–94.
6. Litynski GS. Erich Mühe and the rejection of laparoscopic cholecystectomy (1985): a surgeon ahead of his time. JSLS. 1998;2(4):341–6.

13. Device Development for the Innovative Clinician: Intellectual Property and Regulatory Basics

Jeffrey Ustin and Jeffrey L. Ponsky

This chapter is meant as a primer on device development for the innovative clinician. This is a brief overview with an emphasis on the basics of intellectual property (IP) and regulatory definitions. Other aspects such as selecting and refining needs, reimbursement/business model considerations, and technical development only will be touched upon. An excellent resource for further investigation is *Biodesign: The Process of Innovating Medical Technologies* by Zenios, Makower, and Yock.

Medical device innovation is an involved process that begins with the identification of a need. Subsequently, various approaches to solve the identified problem are considered and weighted. The specific solution is chosen by evaluating the IP space, technologies involved or available, business models, cultural considerations, funding, and regulatory arena. All these factors are important throughout the development process. However, the relative weight of each changes over the development life cycle.

Once an initial need has been identified, the innovator must learn everything there is to know about the problem to be addressed including: (1) the clinical problem (i.e. physiology and pathophysiology involved); (2) market analysis (i.e. how much money is spent on this problem annually, how much growth is anticipated, who is addressing the problem currently); and (3) who will be interested in a solution, including their values, needs, and investments (i.e. patients, physicians, supply chain managers, insurers, etc).

© Springer International Publishing Switzerland 2016   137
S.C. Stain et al. (eds.), *The SAGES Manual Ethics
of Surgical Innovation*, DOI 10.1007/978-3-319-27663-2_13

Brainstorming and Early Development

With this essential information in hand, the innovator can begin brainstorming. At first, all ideas and various approaches are entertained. Each idea can be scored based on its ability to address the underlying problem, how well it will be accepted by the various stakeholders, whether there is IP space in which to innovate (e.g. the idea has been patented already), how mature the technology around the idea is, how complex the anticipated regulatory process would be, and how clean the business approach would be.

It should be obvious that this requires input from people with various expertise. A clinician can provide information from a medical perspective, a business person can analyze the markets and stakeholders, an engineer can identify the current state of the technology, a lawyer can investigate the prior art involved with the IP, and a regulatory expert can evaluate what is likely to be entailed in pursuing permission from the government to market and use what is being created.

While with experience the innovator can become facile with the initial phase of many of these areas, the first time developer needs a great deal of assistance. Most academic institutions have a technology transfer office (TTO). Engagement with the TTO begins with submission of an invention disclosure form (IDF). The IDF asks for basic information about the invention, inventors, market, and IP. The role of the TTO varies from institution to institution. In some cases, it looks for corporate sponsors to fund further research and patenting or to license the proposed technology. More sophisticated TTOs can help incubate an idea by supporting with advanced market anaylsis, performing a customer needs assessment, engaging an IP search, or funding proof of concept prototyping. Most institutions have ownership of any technology that is invented by its employees if the idea was generated through the clinical practice or supported in any fashion by the institution. Thus, the TTO has a great deal of say in what happens with the invention. If the TTO decides not to pursue the invention, the inventor can often form a start-up company and license the technology back from the institution for further development.

If the beginning innovator does not work for an academic institution, there are other options to seek support. Often there is an entrepreneur in the community who can offer further guidance directly or via introduction to somcone knowledgeable about biodesign. Many regions have community-supported incubators that provide guidance and resources early in the development process. Alternatively, most established device manufacturers have a mechanism for engaging innovators. The point of initial contact can be learned via the local representative or simply the company's website.

Intellectual Property Rights

However, before entering any discussion about the innovation, it is important to consider intellectual property basics. The primary mechanism for protecting a medical device is the patent. Most medical device patents are utility patents that describe how the new device does something versus a design patent that can be loosely described as defining how something appears. A patent is granted based on novelty and obviousness. The patent itself is comprised of claims. To be novel, at least one of the claims must be original, never having appeared in any form, ever, worldwide. To meet the second criterion, a typical person working in the field involved with the invention must find the concept to be nonobvious, which can be a very subjective consideration.

Historically, the United States Patent and Trademark Office (USPTO) worked on a first to invent basis. This meant that if two overlapping patents were filed, the inventor who could prove he or she was working on the innovation first won the patent. Now, the USPTO uses a first to file system, meaning regardless of how long someone has been working on a concept, the first patent submitted wins. Patenting can be a very expensive process, easily costing between $5,000–25,000 or more. A much more economical approach is to file a provisional patent. Many times these can be submitted without the assistance of an attorney and cost approximately $200. If an attorney is employed, the provisional patent still only costs on the order of $2000. The provisional patent establishes a priority date. As long as the subsequent full patent meets several requirements, the priority date can be used as the filing date. One requirement is that the full patent be filed within 1 year of the provisional. Failure to do so, sacrifices the priority date. An additional use for the provisional patent is to protect the patentability of an idea when a public disclosure is being made. For clinicians, this occurs when a research project is being published or presented publicly. Filing a provisional patent prior to the disclosure protects the concept, as long as a full patent is filed within a year. Finally, a provisional patent offers an element of protection to the inventor who is need of discussing an idea to move it forward. In this last circumstance, it is also helpful to utilize a non-disclosure agreement that basically states what will be revealed cannot be stolen from the inventor.

The foundation of all IP work is the patent search. This can be completed via the USPTO office or Google patents. Devices are categorized via a system established by the USPTO. It is possible to go search a given category under which the concept being invented exists. All patents in that category can then be examined. A better method is to search for patents that are similar to what is being considered. Make a spreadsheet of all patents uncovered. Then, look at each patent. If it indeed contains similar elements to what is being considered, examine the "referenced by" and "references" category of that patent (both items are included on the first page of the patent). These two contain a list of other patents that are related in at least one element. Add the patents in the "referenced by" and "references" to the spreadsheet and iterate. This is a time-consuming process to do well.

Ultimately, the patent offers some protection against others using a given innovation. However, it does not guarantee the inventor the right to use the innovation in any situation. The right to make and sell an invention is referred to as the freedom to operate. Namely, if the specific innovation is contained in a more general patent, the freedom to operate may not exist.

Prototyping and Regulatory Concerns

By this stage in the process, the goal is to have a specific solution emerging to solve the identified need. Now comes the time for prototyping. It is very useful to generate a first version to hold, touch, and demonstrate to others. This can be created with household items, materials from the local home improvement store, or even 3D printing, which has become readily available. Again, the TTO may be useful in supporting or identifying local machine shops, electronic fabricators, or prototypers to assist.

As the development process continues and a prototype is settled on, attention shifts to regulatory concerns. The regulatory process in the USA is governed by the Food and Drug Administration (FDA) and is largely determined by the type of technology being introduced and the risk posed to the patient.

The FDA mandate to ensure safety and effectiveness of devices comes from an initial Congressional act in 1976, the Medical Device

Amendments Act (MDAA). The MDAA divides devices into three classes based on risk posed. The Safe Medical Devices Act of 1990 further expanded the FDA's regulatory power. The classes at the core of the MDAA determine the degree of the burden of proof for safety/effectiveness.

Class I is a simple device with minimal risk such as a clamp or bandage. Approximately half of all devices are Class I. The vast majority of these require registration, labeling, and a standard quality assurance, but no demonstration of safety or effectiveness via a preclinical or clinical trial.

Class II devices are more complex. Infusion pumps, monitors, and electrosurgical devices are all examples of Class II devices. Class II represents approximately 40 % of all devices. In addition to complying with the general FDA controls, Class II devices have special control requirements including special labeling and post-market surveillance. Market clearance is usually achieved by demonstrating similarity to an existing device, known at the 510(k) pathway.

Class III devices are typically implanted devices such as pacemakers, stents, or intraaortic balloons. These devices nearly always require premarket approval, based on data from a large clinical study demonstrating safety and effectiveness.

Approval Process

The ultimate goal of the approval process from a commercial standpoint is to obtain an indications for use (IFU) statement. The IFU determines what information is included in product packaging and what claims can be made in advertising. Of note, the IFU does not determine, nor does the FDA monitor, how the product is used once approved. Thus, it is common practice to use a device "off-label." This is not illegal. However, as always, the clinician must be sure to remain within the standard of care.

There are three FDA regulatory pathways. Device exemption is used primarily, although not exclusively, for Class I devices. Technically, an exempt device does not require "clearance" to be commercialized. The 510(k) pathway is named after the Federal regulation providing for clearance based on equivalence to prior devices. 510(k) is used most commonly, although not exclusively, for Class II devices.

Finally, premarket approval (PMA) is most often used, although again not exclusively, for Class III devices.

Devices falling under "exempt" status are still required to comply with FDA general controls, such as registering the device and manufacturing facilities, complying with FDA labeling standards, and following FDA guidelines for design and manufacturing (Quality System Regulation, QSR).

The sponsor making a 510(k) submission provides one or more predicate devices for comparison. If the device under evaluation is found to be "substantially equivalent" to the predicate devices, then it may achieve 510(k) clearance. The new device must have the same indication for use, the same technological profile, and no additional safety or effectiveness issues when compared with the predicate device(s). This pathway usually requires bench top or animal testing and only occasionally a human trial. 501(k) devices can combine predicates in an effort to demonstrate safety and effectiveness. The predicate devices must either be exempt or have received 510(k) prior to 1976. No PMA device can be used as a predicate.

The PMA process is understandably the most complicated, costly, and challenging of the three. The PMA centers around a larger clinical trial, much more involved than anything required for the 510(k). The clinical study itself entails tens if not hundreds of patients and often more than one institution. The overall submission includes the results of the clinical study as well as all of the information on quality systems compliance, biocompatibility, engineering testing, failure testing, and shelf life.

The investigational device exemption (IDE) is the mechanism by which devices that have not yet passed the full FDA regulatory process can be used in trials. The first consideration in the IDE process is to determine whether the device poses a significant risk. The Institutional Review Board (IRB) makes this determination where the device is to be tested. If the clinical trial is multi-center, there will likely be multiple IRB submissions. If every IRB agrees there is no significant risk, the device may proceed to trial without an FDA-granted IDE.

IDE requires formal FDA application in which basic information supporting safety is provided. This usually centers on animal testing demonstrating biocompatibility and safety testing, as well as data demonstrating compliance with mechanical, electrical, and sterilization standards. With IDE approval, a device can be used and evaluated under close scrutiny, but it may not be marketed or sold.

One additional category to consider is the Humanitarian Device Exemption (HDE). If a Class III device has a projected market that is fewer than several thousand patients annually, the expected revenue from the device would not support an expensive PMA trial. The HDE seeks to address this market reality. The restrictions on the process are stringent. The developer must demonstrate that it offers a unique solution to the clinical problem and that a standard FDA PMA pathway would not work for its device. Furthermore, unless being used for children, the device can not be sold for profit.

The application process begins with the developer choosing the class in which the device is most likely to fall. The FDA provides assistance on its website to help determine the appropriate class. The submission proceeds and is reviewed by the Office of Device Evaluation. Each pathway is significantly more expensive and challenging than the prior. However, there are strategic reasons, beyond the scope of this chapter, why a more stringent pathway may be preferred.

It is important to note that there has been increasing concern about the FDA approval process, most notably pertaining to 510(k) and HDE processes. The 510(k) issues raised revolve around an explosion in the number of predicates listed and combined in, sometimes, bizarre manners. In 2011, the Institute of Medicine recommended eliminating the 510(k) pathway for fear it did not assure safety or effectiveness. Another line of critique concerning the 510(k) pathway centers on developers making an incremental change to a device to maximize profits. Curfman and Redberg suggest that the cost of the minor improvement and concomitant increase in complexity and cost are not warranted. Likewise, there is concern that the HDE does not demonstrate effectiveness. Critics emphasize the contrast between the FDA process for introducing medical devices and drugs.

A final regulatory consideration is overseas (outside the US, oUS) approval. Australia and Canada are modeled roughly after the European (CE Mark) approach and tend to be the most straightforward. Japan, while well organized, can be cumbersome secondary to translation needs. India, China, Russia, and a conglomerate of South American countries are evolving into important entities given their emerging markets, but they have less developed and often challenging regulatory processes. Finally, overseas trials can be simpler to perform given the more lax regulatory environment. The results from these trials can be used to support FDA applications, if all data are made available. However, typically further studies on United States soil are necessary for FDA clearance.

Funding

The entire discussion is theoretical without funding. Seed funding allows the development of prototypes and supports the basic market analysis and IP efforts described above. Often this money comes from the inventors, the inventor's friends and family, and occasionally local grants. Start-up funding then supports further prototype development, animal testing, early regulatory efforts, and IP work. Typically these funds come from angel investors or some venture capitalists. Further funding rounds then support completion of clinical trials, regulatory approval, and establishment of marketing and sales. These are funded primarily by venture capitalists.

Early rounds of funding are typically in exchange for equity in the company, as opposed to lender debt. Most of these ventures are very high risk and have no cash flow. Therefore, they are not eligible for traditional loans. Instead, the investors take a part of the company in exchange for providing the funding. These investments are very expensive. The cost to the innovator is both in terms of loss of percent ownership and decreased control over the direction and vision of the company. However, this is often what it takes to see a project go from idea to implementation in patient care.

Summary

Surgeons are natural inventors. They are intuitive and highly motivated to improve the care of their patients through constant innovation. It is only natural that they frequently develop new tools to facilitate their mission. It is important that surgeons familiarize themselves with the appropriate channels available and necessary to implement their ideas, and to participate in the clinical and economic benefits of their inventions.

Further Reading

1. Fargen KM, Donald F, David F, McDougall CG, Myers PM, Hirsch JA, Mocco J. The FDA approval process for medical devices: an inherently flawed system or a valuable pathway for innovation? J NeuroIntervent Surg. 2013;5(4):269–75.
2. Institute of Medicine. Medical devices and the public's health: the FDA 510(k) clearance process at 35 years. Washington, DC: National Academies Press; 2011.

3. Curfman GD, Redberg RF. Medical devices–balancing regulation and innovation. N Engl J Med. 2011;365:975–7.
4. 7 Tips for Painless FDA 510(k) Regulatory Submissions. Vincent Crabtree, Ph.D., Regulatory Advisor and Project Manager, StarFish Medical. Blog: mdtmag.com. 11/13/13. Accessed 2 Apr 2015.
5. Zenios SA, Makower J, Yock PG. Biodesign: the process of innovating medical technologies. Cambridge: Cambridge University Press; 2010.
6. Pressman D. Patent it yourself. Berkeley: NOLO Press; 2008.
7. Patent Search Tutorial. Stanford Biodesign Program. http://www.stanford.edu/group/biodesign/patentsearch/inventor.html
8. United States Patent and Trademark Office website. Uspto.gov. (Especially, Patents->Getting Started->Patent Basics and Process Overview. Also, Learning Resources->Resources by Audience->Inventors and Entrepreneurs
9. United States Food and Drug Administration website. Fda.gov. (Especially, Medical Devices->Device Advice: Comprehensive Regulatory Assistance->Overview of Medical Device Regulation
10. Roberts JJ. "First to file" patent law starts today: what it means in plain English. March 18, 2013. https://gigaom.com/2013/03/18/first-to-file-patent-law-starts-today-what-it-means-in-plain-english/. Accessed 4 Apr 2015.

14. Training and Credentialing in New Technologies

Meredith C. Duke and Timothy M. Farrell

A variety of competing forces drive or temper the emergence of new surgical technologies. Patients and providers are motivated to improve clinical outcomes, while regulatory agencies seek to limit risk. Entrepreneurs and industry are market driven, whereas academics may crave notoriety. The degree of alignment or contradiction in these forces can affect how quickly a new technology appears. Once it does, systems for training providers develop and mature variably, and evidence of ultimate clinical effectiveness and appropriate utilization follows.

Measures of New Technologies

There is a careful balance of responsibility between the safety of individuals and the safety of society at large [1]. When a new technology or procedure is proposed, it must be assessed along certain parameters: necessity, safety, evidence-based support of effectiveness, applicability, implementation, and training and credentialing. After the general acceptance of a new technology, it must also stand up to the scrutiny of hindsight. Does it truly live up to its expected value? Each of these stages of new technology introduction is covered in this manual. The purpose of this chapter is to explore the issues of training and credentialing, including ethical aspects involved in those processes.

Responsibility for Training Surgeons in New Technologies

In the United States, the national governing body that evaluates new devices and technologies, and approves their use in practice, is the Center for Devices and Radiological Health branch of the US Food and Drug

© Springer International Publishing Switzerland 2016   147
S.C. Stain et al. (eds.), *The SAGES Manual Ethics*
of Surgical Innovation, DOI 10.1007/978-3-319-27663-2_14

Administration (FDA). Included in device approval is the review and approval of training programs proposed for new technologies. The FDA itself does not specifically create, modify, or monitor the content of training programs or educational methods utilized [2]. Therefore, implementation and education of surgeons, particularly practicing surgeons, falls to the responsibility of the individual surgeons themselves, often with the assistance of professional societies and the oversight of local institutions. Professional societies, such as SAGES, play a vital role in expanding and analyzing the body of evidence to clarify best practices and also to guide appropriate training and credentialing of surgeons.

Applicability of New Technologies and Procedures

With the emergence of therapeutic laparoscopy in the 1980s, there was enthusiasm from patients, providers, and industry. Laparoscopic cholecystectomy was a new, state-of-the-art procedure then, and today it has clear applicability for all modern general surgeons. As laparoscopy has matured and the procedures have become more complex, it has become less clear who should be performing these procedures. Nationally, surgeons began asking in the 1990s whether these more advanced procedures fell under the domain of generalists or trained specialists. While patients in general were lured by the tangible benefits of laparoscopy, each surgeon took a personal stance on the necessity of the skill set, and their ability to acquire it.

Local institutions continue to control credentialing, while national organizations like SAGES have been inspired to take a proactive stance regarding training in new technologies and techniques. The society's educational mission has evolved in a way that has been very fruitful. This era was marked by the creation of informal mini fellowships initially, and this effort grew into the formation of the Fellowship Council, which now has national purview over the formal 1–2 year surgical fellowship programs [3].

Implementation of New Technologies at the Institutional Level

As stated before, the FDA is charged with the evaluation of new device safety and approval for marketing, and this approval includes consideration of an appropriate training process. However, the specifics of training are not defined in detail by the FDA. Therefore, the creation of training curricula, metrics of performance, and benchmarks for competency often fall to professional organizations like SAGES, which are comprised of members interested in utilizing the new technology.

SAGES has long-published clinical practice and credentialing guidelines, and in 2012 SAGES created a Technology and Value Assessment Committee (TAVAC). Since monitoring of early implementation of new technologies sometimes identifies suboptimal or unexpected outcomes of those technologies, the SAGES Guidelines Committee and TAVAC review and publish statements on a regular basis, to support active modification of practice patterns and training paradigms [4].

Despite guidelines provided by national organizations, each individual institution is ultimately responsible for evaluating, approving, and monitoring the introduction of new devices. The level of formality in this process varies by institution. Some create multidisciplinary committees charged with this task, while others frequently employ informal implementation programs. The makeup of these groups varies widely and may only include peers or a division chair. There is a potential for conflict of interest, and inter-physician conflict, when physicians from different disciplines are seeking approval for the same or similar technologies [5]. This is a situation when it may be helpful to have a formal committee that oversees and approves implementation, credentialing, and also monitoring of early outcomes to ensure safety and quality patient care.

Training Paradigms for Postgraduate Trainees and Practicing Surgeons

During acquisition of new knowledge and skills, learners need access to experts, places to practice, and time. Trainees and practicing surgeons have varying challenges in achieving such access. Valid educational interventions for new techniques and technologies are needed for both trainees and surgeons in practice. Such interventions should include a curriculum with structured teaching, which is individualized to the specific needs of learners at different places in the educational process. It is necessary to verify the acquisition of knowledge and skills by ensuring attainment of benchmark levels using validated assessment tools [6].

For both trainees and practicing surgeons, preceptors are a vital component of the educational environment. They serve to provide real-time feedback and to verify achievement of benchmarks as the surgeon acquires component skills. Ultimately, preceptors serve to safeguard patients during a learner's implementation of a new technology in a real-world setting such as the operating room.

Faculty members serve the preceptor role in the academic training environment of residency and fellowship. For practicing surgeons, access to preceptors is more difficult. Some may have to rely upon a partner with the given expertise. Otherwise, time away from practice is necessary to allow a validated course of fellowship.

Proctors are also often employed during the introduction of new technologies. Preceptors actively participate in the procedure and the education process, while proctors tend to be supervisors or independent evaluators. A threshold of proctored cases is often required prior to independent application of a new technology or procedure. This number is often arbitrary and not based on solid evidence of effectiveness [7]. For procedures that are rare and have a steep learning curve, evidence-based competency thresholds are not a realistic goal.

A training program must identify standards upon which to monitor physicians' outcomes when implementing new technologies and techniques, and it must have a reliable system of reporting. Standards need to incorporate patient selection, technical skills, and clinical outcomes. Outcomes are important to monitor because they can drive curriculum change within the training program and also factor into the important issues of credentialing and remediation for the individual surgeon [6].

Credentialing

There are bodies that have been established to ensure patient safety at the level of health care institutions (The Joint Commission, NSQIP, hospital privileging committees). However, the sensitivity to variations in patient outcomes related to implementation of new technologies or techniques will be limited due to the sampling methods and the aggregated nature of the measures. Monitoring systems that derive from educational programs and professional societies are more likely to be sensitive to important outcomes and can drill down to the individual provider more easily.

In residency or fellowship training, the teaching faculty is responsible for credentialing a given learner. Program directors and chairs recognize that when they sign a training certificate they are attesting to the competency of that graduate with their reputations. If that is not enough, training programs are also overseen by credentialing bodies, like the Accreditation Council for Graduate Medical Education (ACGME) or the

Fellowship Council, which can alter program certifications if educators are not fulfilling their obligations.

For those practicing surgeons who are implementing new techniques or technologies, the educational process is typically driven by the continuing education offerings of professional societies. These societies include faculty members who teach residents and fellows regularly and who are committed to the training paradigm, including the use of validated curricula, structured and individualized teaching, use of assessment tools with benchmarks, and monitoring. Like residency and fellowship programs, professional societies have oversight of their educational activities, in this case through the Accreditation Council for Continuing Medical Education (ACCME).

For emerging technologies, there are multiple layers to the degree of additional training and credentialing necessary. This spectrum can range from board certification/eligibility to external monitoring through a center of excellence. Intermediate options include gaining familiarity, self-assessment and peer review, training courses, and ultimately fellowship training. The level of training and credentialing necessary should be congruent with the degree of technology change and the risk incumbent to the patient [8].

The best monitoring comes when individual surgeons commit to the use of surgeon-specific registries so that outcomes can be compared with those of peers [7]. The American College of Surgeons (ACS) and several specialty organizations are offering these resources to their members. In most cases, use is voluntary but may be tied to certain program certifications that are important to the individual surgeon. It is clear that, before long, detailed surgeon-specific outcomes tracking will be ubiquitous.

Examples of New Technologies in Practice

When introducing new technologies, there will always be supporters and adversaries. The supporters have a vision of improved patient care, while the adversaries see the potential increased risk. Even when evidence proves that a new method is safe and superior, there is lag time in introduction and implementation. Reasons for this include the desire for stability and reproducibility, as well as aversion to change. Grace Hopper, a Rear Admiral for the US Navy, was credited with saying, "Humans are allergic to change. They love to say, 'We've always done it this way'" [9]. Surgeons are no different. For many who have trained and practiced a tried-and-true method, they find little motivation for change and they highlight the potential for increased risk.

Surgeons have always had to assess new technologies and techniques and then make decisions about whether to assimilate them into practice. Every day a patient-by-patient evaluation of the tools at their disposal is performed, and surgeons have to choose the appropriate application to achieve optimal results. The individual surgeon's choice whether to employ the laparoscopic approach to cholecystectomy in 1989–1993 was an exercise of this dichotomy of thinking, and the lessons learned bolstered the argument for each side of the laparoscopy argument. Since the disorganized emergence of laparoscopic cholecystectomy, the surgical community has recognized the need to improve these processes, and it has done so actively.

Laparoscopic Cholecystectomy

Laparoscopic cholecystectomy was a dramatic paradigm shift driven by surgeon innovators and industry partners. However, it was the sudden demand from patients and referring providers that exposed the inadequacies of the educational system for surgeons in practice. While some surgeons were interested in the potential benefits of laparoscopic surgery, patients recognized the value of smaller incisions, less pain, and shorter recovery time. The technology advancement was alluring to patients, and many surgeons will remember patients asking for "laser surgery."

As surgeons began to encounter increasing patient demand, many saw value in marketing themselves and this new technology. In some cases, billboards and other nontraditional methods were employed by private surgeons. Those in academia were also aware of the opportunity to promote their careers around this new technology. Scientific manuscripts and skills courses rapidly emerged in this era.

Industry was supportive of science and education; laparoscopy was a completely new and untapped market. There was a race to dominate market share, and as the potential for return on investment continued to climb, industry drove research and development.

The situation put all these stakeholders in alignment, and so patients, surgeons, and industry put the demand for laparoscopy out of balance with the supply of trained practitioners. This situation caused the training model to depend on weekend courses, self-study, and new practitioners educating partners on their newly acquired skill set. For the most part, laparoscopic cholecystectomy emerged ahead of the evidence.

Table 14.1. Published rate of bile duct injury in early laparoscopic cholecystectomy.

Study	Bile duct injury rate (%)
Deziel (1993)	0.6
Wherry (1994)	0.52
Wherry (1996)	0.47
Nuzzo (2005)	0.4
Waage (2006)	0.4
Steady state rate	0.4

Data from Marohn M (2011) Fear during the routine lap chole: the bile duct might be/is injured. Video presented at SAGES 2011. Symposium Managing Complications and Re-operations

Scientific sessions and publications were the first formal outcomes reporting. Given its focus in endoscopy, SAGES was involved early in this process, delivering information about the efficacy and safety of this new technology. It became clear early on that bile duct injury rates were at least twice that of open cholecystectomy [10–13] (Table 14.1). With this evidence, SAGES modified the curriculum and focused scientific sessions and publications on the issue of improving safety and limiting complications. SAGES sponsored national and regional courses, and in 1990 it published the first guideline on biliary tract surgery. This guideline has been revised every few years since then. Following these SAGES-inspired improvements in training, the bile duct injury rate for laparoscopic cholecystectomy improved, though it has plateaued at 0.4 %, which is still higher than that associated with open cholecystectomy [12]. In spite of this information, patients are willing to accept this increased risk in exchange for the tangible benefits—better cosmesis, decreased pain, decreased length of stay, and earlier return to activities of daily living.

In retrospect, it is clear that laparoscopic cholecystectomy could not have happened without the bold surgeons and industry partners who drove it to common practice. However, the method of dissemination of this technology was not ideal. SAGES recognized this discrepancy, and as a consequence, the importance of its educational mission and the methods by which to accomplish have become more clear.

Advanced Laparoscopy

The emergence of advanced laparoscopy for foregut, colorectal, and other procedures defined a second wave of new laparoscopic technology that affected general surgery. Patient demand was still a driving force as was surgeon marketing and industry interest.

The training model for teaching advanced laparoscopy differed from laparoscopic cholecystectomy in that it saw the emergence of a select few experts who had mastered the technique and who were capable and motivated to educate and teach these advanced procedures. Instead of a reliance on weekend courses, these leaders drove the training model forward by offering informal mini fellowships and eventually formal 1–2 year fellowships for surgeons desiring specialization in these methods.

The surgical community was scrutinizing the evidence and publishing comparative studies addressing whether clinical and quality-of-life outcomes were equivalent or better. In addition, experts were writing about complication reduction, defining learning curves, and identifying volume/outcomes relationships. The message to the surgical community was clear—these techniques and technologies require formal training [14].

SAGES emerged to fill the training gap for practicing surgeons and trainees. The society took a more proactive stance in the training model compared to what had occurred with laparoscopic cholecystectomy. This included an integrated strategy—running national and regional courses, creating practice and credentialing guidelines, and driving the formalization of fellowships. Some surgeons chose to acquire the skill set, whereas others narrowed their practices or acquired specialty-trained partners.

SAGES inspired formation of the MIS Fellowship Council, later renamed the Fellowship Council (FC). The creation of the FC improved the match process for applicants and programs, and it later developed a system for program accreditation. The FC also collectively bargained for fellowship funding, and it later created a free-standing foundation called the Foundation for Surgical Fellowships (FSF) to ensure ethical and unbiased distribution of donated educational funds [3]. Fellowships have become the accepted training model for advanced laparoscopy, and the potential for conflicts of interest with industry have been minimized by standardized funding paradigms.

Looking back, it is clear that technology and procedure development around advanced laparoscopy expanded the market for surgical therapy for common conditions. More patients became interested in surgery because surgeons were able to accomplish procedures with equivalent or improved results with smaller incisions and shorter recovery times.

The success of laparoscopy for patients and providers alike has stimulated surgeons in practice to stay abreast of new technologies in order to maintain relevance as modern surgeons.

SAGES educational focus and adherence to ethical business practices have put the society in a position of prominence and influence with the governing bodies of American Surgery as they restructure curricula and define credentialing in areas of new procedures and technology.

Laparoscopic Adjustable Gastric Banding

The emergence of adjustable gastric banding deserves special attention. This procedure and associated technologies were popularized outside the United States due to perceived low operative risk and reversibility. American companies invested heavily to bring adjustable gastric banding to the USA. There were enthusiastic physicians looking to diversify their practices and to satisfy patient demand. Once again, the driving forces were aligned, but this procedure required more significant industry presence due to FDA implant approval and training mandates. Interaction between surgical experts and industry partners was necessary to drive early education, and courses were supported by industry funding.

The laparoscopic gastric banding market exploded and so did the literature surrounding bariatric surgery. Gastric banding was compared to both medical management and other operations previously offered, namely the gastric bypass. Early data supported a significantly lower short-term mortality rate and reasonable success. Much of the stigma surrounding bariatric surgery was lifted thanks to innovative marketing and industry influence. Unfortunately, as the literature bore out, the morbidity and revision rate of gastric banding were much greater than previously appreciated [15].

There were a number of factors that drove the popularity of gastric band placement, despite literature arguing against widespread application. Patients found the reversibility of the procedure appealing. Surgeons found it to be a technically simpler operation that did not require fellowship training. Industry was motivated to aggressively push implementation following the "first-mover" strategy—a simple theory that argues being the first to a market provides an actual and potential benefit against rivals. One can achieve brand loyalty, product familiarity, market share, and distribution benefits.

The gastric band experience illustrates the importance of timing regarding new technology introduction. "Introduction of a new procedure or an emerging technology should be timed carefully and strike a balance between waiting for sufficient data to support its use and the health care needs of patients while data are being collected. Late introduction of a new modality may deprive the patients of adequate or state-of-the-art care" [6]. In the case of the gastric band, the balance was outweighed by the patient, industry, and surgeon push for application and the inability to maintain patience for data collection and analysis. Experience gained from the gastric band motivated our governing bodies to look more closely into who can and should provide which services, and qualifications necessary to achieve this ability. Through the collaboration of the ACS, the American Society of Metabolic and Bariatric Surgeons (ASMBS), and SAGES, co-endorsed bariatric surgery guidelines and rules for bariatric centers of excellence have been accepted. The need for continuous monitoring of individual and national outcomes via registries is highlighted.

Summary

There is a constant enthusiasm for innovation driving surgeons, patients, and industry partners to develop and disseminate novel treatments and devices. This drive must be tempered by consideration of uncertain risks, unproven benefits, and increased costs. The government, through the FDA, assures that new devices do not pose undue risk at rollout, but the true measure of safety, efficacy, and cost effectiveness requires time and comparative study. Establishing clinical indications, guidelines, and best practices is most effectively done by professional organizations, like SAGES, which have the resources to perform critical review and refinement during early implementation, with attention to the possibility of conflict of interest.

Professional organizations like SAGES will continue to guide dissemination of new techniques and procedures through their educational missions and infrastructure. As courses and formal fellowships were developed when the need for better education of practicing surgeons and trainee surgeons was identified during the emergence of advanced minimally invasive gastrointestinal surgery, new technologies such as robotics will continue to drive critical assessment and the formation of structured training pathways under SAGES auspices.

It is paramount that SAGES maintains its leadership role in innovating, validating, training, and credentialing new technologies in gastrointestinal and endoscopic surgery, with the purpose of ensuring safe and effective implementation, and guaranteeing the primacy of patient welfare over all other considerations.

References

1. Riskin DJ, Longaker MT, Gertner M, Krummel TM. Innovation in surgery: a historical perspective. Ann Surg. 2006;244:686–93.
2. US Food and Drug Administration. About the Center for Devices and Radiological Health. http://www.fda.gov/AboutFDA/CentersOffices/OfficeofMedicalProductsand Tobacco/CDRH/ (2015). Accessed 17 Apr 2015.
3. The Fellowship Council. About the Fellowship Council. https://fellowshipcouncil.org/about/ (2015). Accessed 22 Mar 2015.
4. Oleynikov D. Evolving responsibility for SAGES – TAVAC. video presented at SAGES 2014. Symposium Ethics of Innovation. 2014.
5. Strong VE, Forde KA, MacFadyen BV, et al. Ethical considerations regarding the implementation of new technologies and techniques in surgery. Surg Endosc. 2014;28(8):2272–6. doi:10.1007/s00464-014-3644-1.
6. Sachdeva A, Russell T. Safe introduction of new procedures and emerging technologies in surgery: education, credential, and privileging. Surg Clin N Am. 2007;87:853–66.
7. Stefanidis D, Fanelli RD, Price R, Richardson W. SAGES guidelines for the introduction of new technology and techniques. Surg Endosc. 2014;28(8):2257–71. doi:10.1007/s00464-014-3587-6.
8. Pellegrini CA, Sachdeva AK, Johnson KA. Accreditation of education institutes by the American College of Surgeons: a new program following an old tradition. Bull Am Coll Surg. 2006;91(3):9–12.
9. Schieber P. The wit and wisdom of Grace Hopper. OCLC Newsletter. March/April. 1987.
10. Barkun JS. Randomised controlled trial of laparoscopic versus mini cholecystectomy. The McGill Gallstone Treatment Group. Lancet. 1992;340:1116–9.
11. Williams Jr LF, Chapman WC, Bonau RA, et al. Comparison of laparoscopic cholecystectomy with open cholecystectomy in a single center. Am J Surg. 1993;165(4):459–65.
12. Club SS. A prospective analysis of 1518 laparoscopic cholecystectomies. N Engl J Med. 1991;324:1073–8.
13. Marohn M. Fear during the routine lap chole: the bile duct might be/is injured. video presented at SAGES 2011. Symposium Managing Complications and Re-operations. 2011.
14. Wexner SD, Eisen GM, Simmang C. Principles of privileging and credentialing for endoscopy and colonoscopy. Surg Endosc. 2002;16:367–9.
15. Himpens J, Cadiere JB, Bazi M, et al. Long-term outcomes of laparoscopic adjustable gastric banding. Arch Surg. 2011;146(7):802–7. doi:10.1001/archsurg.2011.45.

15. Informed Consent and Surgical Innovation

Lelan F. Sillin, Arthur L. Rawlings,
and Phillip P. Shadduck

The goal of the informed consent process is to lead a patient or a potential research subject to make an educated and voluntary choice for or against a treatment pathway or research participation. There is robust literature on informed consent for treatment and for research. There is less on informed consent in the context of surgical innovation. The goal of this chapter is to review informed consent for clinical treatment and for research involving human subjects and then examine it in the context of surgical innovation. There are several aspects of informed consent that can be discussed in detail—the process, decisional capacity, coercion, establishment of trust, etc.—but the focus here will be on the informational content as this will help highlight how informed consent for surgical innovation is similar and different from the other two categories, and allow some guidelines to be expressed.

Informed Consent for Clinical Practice

The history of informed consent is largely a legal history that is focused on clinical treatment. There are elements, however, of even the earliest case in Anglo-Saxon jurisprudence, which hint of the controversies involved in clinical innovation and research. In the 1767 case of Slater v. Baker & Stapleton, the patient had a fractured leg which had been initially treated by another physician. Mr. Slater went to Dr. Baker to have his dressing changed. With only permission to change the dressing, Dr. Baker, with the assistance of Dr. Stapleton, refractured the leg and placed it in an experimental device which they believed would both straighten the fractured bone and improve healing. The patient successfully

© Springer International Publishing Switzerland 2016   159
S.C. Stain et al. (eds.), *The SAGES Manual Ethics*
of Surgical Innovation, DOI 10.1007/978-3-319-27663-2_15

sued for breach of contract, similar to the current day concept of lack of consent, and for treating him contrary to the standard of practice [1].

In 1914, in the case of Schloendorff v. Society of New York Hospital, Judge Cardoza, later to be an Associate Justice on the United States (US) Supreme Court, famously wrote "every human being of adult years and sound mind has a right to determine what shall be done with his own body; and a surgeon who performs an operation without his patient's consent commits an assault for which he is liable in damages." The opinion went on to say that the surgeon performed treatment that the patient had not authorized. The surgeon should have informed her of the risks and alternatives involved in the treatment prior to taking any action other than that which was authorized. This case established the principle of **patient autonomy** as one of the fundamental tenets of informed consent [1].

Three cases [Natanson v. Kline (1960); Canterbury v. Spence (1972); Truman v. Thomas (1980)] further established the principle of patient autonomy and the requirement of the treating physician to disclose the material risks and benefits of the treatment to the patient prior to starting that care. Also, the risks of the treatment are to be disclosed from the patient's point of view, not the physician's point of view. This discussion of risks must also include the risks of refusal of treatment [1].

These fundamental legal principles are now firmly established in American law. Virtually all states recognize the right of patients to receive information about their medical condition, the treatment options, risks, expected outcomes, and prognosis associated with their condition. Failure to obtained informed consent for nonemergencies may be a civil (negligence) and/or criminal (battery) offense.

The principle of patient autonomy as the basis for informed consent is supported in the process of consent by three basic elements: disclosure, understanding, and patient decision. **Disclosure** is the dissemination of the information that the patient has a right to know. The disclosure can include, but is not limited to, the diagnosis, the current condition, the expected course with and without treatment, the specific treatment recommendations, a description of any recommended procedure, the definition and probability of success, the risks and benefits of each option, and finally "any other information generally provided to patients in this situation by other qualified physicians" [1].

Three different standards are used to assess the adequacy of the disclosed information. The first is the *reasonable physician standard*, which is the disclosure of information that a typical physician would believe is adequate. The second, the *reasonable patient standard*, is what a typical patient would need to know to be an informed participant in the decision-making process. This is the most widely applied standard in the USA. The third, the *subjective standard*, is the disclosure of the information that this particular patient would need to know in order to make an informed decision. This is discussed in the literature, but has not yet been applied in any state or in any specific case.

The second major element of the informed consent process is **understanding**. It is important for the treating physician to provide all of the requisite information. It is equally important that the patient understands the information. This places a responsibility on the physician to be sure that the patient understands what is being communicated. The level of understanding needed for a proper consent is difficult to elucidate as it varies from situation to situation even with the same patient. Suffice it to say that the patient must have enough of an understanding of the risks, benefits, and alternatives to treatment to make an autonomous decision.

The third element of the informed consent process is **decisional capacity**, which is distinct from competence. Competence is a legal status. Everyone is assumed to be competent until a court of law determines him or her to be incompetent. Decisional capacity is a functional status—it requires that a patient have the ability to understand relevant information, to appreciate the medical situation, to engage in rational deliberation, and to be able to communicate their decision. This can be determined by a medical professional as is done daily in clinic settings when physicians discuss with their patients medical conditions and treatment options.

The final component of the informed consent is that the decision maker must authorize the procedure or treatment plan freely. Persuasion by the physician may be appropriate; coercion is not.

Informed consent for treatment is not without its problems, limitations, or challenges. The surgeon may have poor communication skills, be uncertain of the appropriate treatment plan, be unwilling to alarm the patient, or even be anxious about the situation itself. The patient may also be a source of limitation for a number of reasons including limited capacity to understand, inattentiveness to the explanations given, distractions by various factors including the illness itself, an unwillingness to listen to the information being presented, anxiety, and other factors. Decisional capacity may wax and wane as a result of many factors including the illness. Religious and cultural issues also may affect the decisional capacity of the patient. These must be recognized, acknowledged, and dealt with. This may require participation by family members, clergy, other religious or cultural authorities, or even other outside assistance. None of these factors erase the need to engage in the process.

Finally, it must always be remembered that a reasonable patient may refuse the recommended therapy or procedure [1].

In summary, informed consent for clinical treatment has three basic components. The individual making the decision should:

1. Have sufficient detail disclosed by the surgeon about the disease, treatment recommendations, and alternatives including the risks and benefits of each, and a description of the course of the disease with no treatment
2. Have the capacity to make the decision
3. Be able to express their decision so a pathway forward can be agreed upon by the physician and the patient

Informed Consent for Research

Informed consent for research involving human subjects is different from that for clinical treatment, just as research is different from treatment. The goal of clinical treatment is to apply medical knowledge to the benefit of the individual patient. The goal of research is to generate generalized medical knowledge, which may benefit society but may not necessarily benefit the individual research subject. Consequently, the patient needs additional protections when being asked to be a research subject and when participating in a research project.

The recent history of the development of informed consent for research involving human subjects grew out of the atrocities committed by the Nazis before and during World War II. The first document from this era to specifically address the consent process required for using human beings as experimental subjects was the Nuremberg Code developed in 1947. The Code is a document with legal intent that specifically articulated the required elements for the consent for participation of an experimental subject. It requires that the consent be voluntary and informed, and that the individual understand the information presented and have decisional capacity. The first and major principle that the Code emphasizes is that "the voluntary consent of the human subject is absolutely essential" [2]. It is understandable that, in the aftermath of the experiments of World War II, human autonomy would be the central focus of ethics applied to research.

In 1964, the World Medical Association formulated the Declaration of Helsinki that sought to articulate an ethical code to be used by investigators for medical research involving human subjects [3]. It has been revised several times and still serves as a foundational document in research ethics. However, in 1966 Dr. Henry Beecher published an article in the New England Journal of Medicine, which evaluated several articles published over the preceding 10 years in prominent journals and by reputable investigators. His detailed analysis of these studies indicated that each of them violated a number of the principles enumerated in both the Nuremberg Code and the Declaration of Helsinki. The Beecher article revealed the power that physicians have over their patients, and it exposed the potential conflict of interest between the physicians' duty to treat their patients' illness and their role as an investigator. It reinforced the practical need for engaging in a rigorous informed consent process [1].

Congress in 1974, responding to continued revelations of medical research which did not meet the standards articulated in the Nuremberg Code or the Declaration of Helsinki, established the National Commission for the Protection of Human Subjects of Biomedical Research and Behavioral Research. The commission was charged with identifying the ethical principles involved in using human subjects. The resulting work is known as the Belmont Report, published in 1979 [4]. While it is not law, the Belmont Report forms the basis for the uniform set of regulations—the Federal Policy for the Protection of Human Subjects at the Office for Human Research Protections. It identifies three basic ethical principles central to human subject research: respect for persons, beneficence, and justice. These principles are to be applied to research involving human beings in three primary areas: informed consent, assessment of risks and benefits, and the selection of subjects.

The **principle of respect for persons** demands voluntary informed consent of the participant and the protection of vulnerable persons, especially those with diminished autonomy such as children. The **principle of beneficence** requires that the proposed study seek to maximize the benefits for the participants and to minimize the harms or potential harms to them. Finally, the **principle of justice** requires that there be appropriate selection of subjects and that those populations less likely to benefit from the research not be over represented in the study population.

Because patients are potentially more vulnerable when asked to be research subjects than when they are asked for which treatment option they want, they need more information to give informed consent for research than for the clinical treatment of their disease. The Belmont Report and its implications require that consent be totally voluntary and fully informed as an absolute for participation in human research. It requires that subjects being asked to participate are informed that this is a research project, that they may refuse to participate, and that they may withdraw from the study at any time. They are able to do these things without any penalty or threat to their continued medical treatment [4]. These requirements and others in the Belmont Report and its successors have been universally adopted in the USA. They have been formalized and are generally protected through an institution-based structure known as the Institutional Review Board (IRB). The consent document for research has a long list of well-defined elements enumerating these requirements and protections that must be included in the document presented to the patient.

Thus, the informed consent process for research differs substantially from that required for clinical treatment. The process for research focuses on the experimental study and its effects on and its implications for the human subject. The consent process for clinical treatment seeks to inform the patient about how an intervention will address their disease or condition and the risks and benefits associated with that intervention.

Informed Consent for Innovation

Attempts to define and classify surgical innovation, particularly in its relationship to research, have proven to be challenging [5–7]. The two polar opposites of classic clinical practice and classic research are rather distinct. Surgical innovation, however, sits along the continuum of these polar opposites of treatment and research. The Belmont Report itself recognized that "the distinction between research and practice is blurred partly because both often occur together (as in research designed to evaluate a therapy) and partly because notable departures from standard practice are often called 'experimental' when the terms 'experimental' and 'research' are not carefully defined" [4]. It goes on to state that "When a clinician departs in a significant way from standard or accepted practice, the innovation does not, in and of itself, constitute research. The fact that a procedure is 'experimental', in the sense of new, untested, or different, does not automatically place it in the category of research." However, the report also notes that "Research and practice may be carried on together when research is designed to evaluate the safety and efficacy of a therapy" [4]. It comments that "such activity should not be the source of any confusion about the need for review," and that the "general rule is that if there is any element of research in an activity, that activity should undergo review for the protection of human subjects" [4]. Surgeons, and perhaps all interventionists, have long known that innovation is an integral part of their craft and, hence, spend time in that continuum between clinical treatment and research [5–7]. How informed consent is to be carried out in that arena is worthy of discussion.

The surgical community has been working toward an understanding of when innovations in surgical practice become a research endeavor so that patients can be given the protections mandated for human research subjects when appropriate. However, it is not clear how many of the surgeon innovators are engaged in the discussion. The University of Virginia Center for Biomedical Ethics surveyed surgeons who had published articles about innovative surgery. Fourteen of the 21 surgical authors responding to the survey identified their project as research yet only 6 of those 14 obtained IRB review. Only 7 of the 21 authors noted the innovative nature of the procedure in their consent discussions with their patients [8]. In a subsequent article, the same group surveyed 665 surgeons, and only about half of the surgeons identified the statement "comparing a new technique to the existing standard of care, retrospectively" qualified as research [9]. This is a soberingly sad commentary on our understanding of research. These data provoked Bracken-Roche et al. to opine that "A key challenge to consider is whether, or how well, patients are informed and understand that their therapy is innovative and may involve unknown risks and benefits" [10]. They concluded that surgeon innovators appear to generally inform their patients about the innovative nature of the procedure but that they do not necessarily include this information in the consent document [10].

Concerns about the performance of surgical treatments of unproven worth without a proper consent have been expressed by others. McKneally writes "Nonvalidated surgical procedures are being 'smuggled' past RCTs and IRBs, our societal checkpoints for innovation, in the same way that minor variations in surgical practice have always been introduced, without institutional review" [5]. Lantos worries that the consent process for innovative procedures is motivated largely by concerns about malpractice litigation rather than concern for patient protection, and he opines that adverse events and outcomes are under reported [11]. Both Ivy and Fost express apprehension that these attitudes and behaviors are even more prevalent in the private practice setting [12, 13].

Bracken-Roche and colleagues noted that the way a particular surgical innovation is framed to patients and colleagues may have important implications. "When characterized as research, innovation is subject to stringent regulatory oversight that includes specific provisions to ensure that participants have given a free and informed consent." But they warned "this oversight is bypassed when innovation is labeled as clinical care, which may have serious consequences for the protection of patients and their exercise of autonomy" [10].

In 2008, in response to the increasing discussions in conceptual ethics and the medical literature, particularly the observations of Reitsma and Moreno [8, 9], the Society of University Surgeons (SUS) appointed a task force that published a position statement on the ethical and practical framework for managing surgical innovations [14]. The SUS noted that "surgical innovation in itself is not problematic," and it is in some sense necessary, but that "the absence of any organized oversight or mechanism to protect patients from becoming an unwitting research subject is, however, problematic" [14].

Research was defined by the) SUS as "a systematic investigation, including development, testing, and evaluation, designed to develop or contribute to generalized knowledge." So if the basic intent is to disseminate information—publicize or publish it—then it should be considered research. Under these circumstances, the informed consent process must meet all of the IRB requirements and adhere to the principles of human subject research in the manual <u>Protecting Study Volunteers in Research</u> [14].

Variation was defined by the SUS as a minor modification of the surgical procedure that does not have a reasonable expectation of increasing the risk to the patient. The implications were that the informed consent here includes a complete description of the critical elements of the proposed procedure, but that "specific details, including the minor variation(s), need not be routinely described and are left to the surgeon's discretion" [14].

Innovation, however, was defined as "modifications of existing procedures that incorporate new or unusual surgical techniques, approaches, or methods which made them appreciably distinct from the standard of care." The SUS recognizes that innovations may be of various types— the response to a specific clinical situation, an attempt to improve outcomes, or the testing of a new idea, technique, instrument or device [14]. The innovation may differ from currently accepted local practice, the outcomes of which have not been described and may entail risk to the patient. It may be an ad hoc development, or it may be a more systematic approach that may ultimately meet criteria for human subject research. They went on to say that "if the procedure is not described in US surgical textbooks its novelty should be part of the informed consent process, even if it is common practice in other parts of the world" [14]. Though all the specifics are not spelled out, the SUS expressed that more information should be given to the patient undergoing a procedure where innovation is involved than if innovation is not involved. That information falls short of what is needed to consent for research, but is more than needed for treatment within the accepted standard of care.

In their systematic review of the literature on the ethics of surgical innovation, Bracken-Roche et al. found that the literature identified four major points of tension: the use of biasing/biased terminology to characterize innovation, patient vulnerability, the relationship between the surgeon innovator and the patient, and practices related to consent and disclosure [10]. Their findings corroborated the more focused study by Lee Char and colleagues from the University of California, San Francisco [15]. Bracken-Roche and Lee Char both found that surgeons and patients overwhelmingly favored special consent and disclosure in the context of innovation. Patients, in particular, wanted information about the novel nature of the procedure, the known risks and benefits, and the acknowledgment of potentially unknown risks and benefits. Most importantly and quite specifically, the patients wanted to know if the surgeon was performing the procedure for the first time [15].

Given the discussion above, some guidelines can be set forth. First, informed consent in the setting of innovation should include full disclosure. This is to be done before the procedure if the innovation is planned and afterwards if it was an ad hoc addition to the standard of care. Secondly, the discussion should include a review of the known outcomes of the innovation or an acknowledgment that the results are unknown at the time, if that is the case. Finally, the intent of the innovation should serve as a criterion for whether full IRB approval is needed. If the intent of the innovation is to improve on a particular person's care or to apply known medical knowledge to a specific situation, IRB approval is likely not needed. If, however, the intent of innovation is to expand general medical knowledge, to promote, publish, or patent this particular innovation, then IRB approval is likely needed. In this regard, the SUS position statement concluded with a sober reminder for surgical innovators that, in the context of innovation, "any omission of such discussion arguably involves deception and violates patient autonomy-based rights to submit to care and could create potential liability for surgeons and their institutions" [14].

Conclusion

Surgical innovation exists in the continuum between clinical practice and research. It has components of both—applying known medical knowledge to a particular patient's condition while also seeking to expand medical knowledge and improving care. For this reason, the informed consent process for innovation requires more discussion with the patient about the procedure, not less. Truthfulness, integrity, transparency, and patience are essential ingredients for engaging in this important process. Institutional Review Boards are designed to protect human subjects in research, and while not all innovation is research, it may be appropriate and prudent to have an IRB make that determination if there is any question as to whether a particular innovation is research or not. This independent determination should be sought by surgeon innovators when appropriate, not for the primary purpose of avoiding ethical or legal entanglements, but in order to ensure both optimal patient care and minimal potential harm.

References

1. Grimm DA. Informed consent for all! No exceptions. New Mexico Law Rev. 2007; 37:39–83.
2. The Nuremberg Code, U.S. National Institutes of Health, Office of Human Subjects Research. http://www.hhs.gov/ohrp/archive/nurcode.html
3. World Medical Association Declaration of Helsinki: ethical principles for medical research involving human subjects (revised October 2013). http://www.wma.net/en/30publications/10policies/b3/
4. The Belmont Report. http://www.hhs.gov/ohrp/humansubjects/guidance/belmont.html
5. McKneally MF. Ethical problems in surgery: innovations leading to unforeseen complication. World J Surg. 1999;23:786–8.
6. Riskin DL, Longaker MT, Gertner M, Krummel TM. Innovation in surgery: a historical perspective. Ann Surg. 2006;244:686–93.
7. Barkun JS, Aronson JK, Feldman LS, Maddern GJ, Strasberg SM, et al. Evaluation and stages of surgical innovations. Lancet. 2009;374:1089–96.
8. Reitsma RA, Moreno JD. Ethical regulation for innovative surgery: the last frontier? J Am Coll Surg. 2002;194:792–801.
9. Reitsma RA, Moreno JD. Ethics of innovative surgery: US surgeons' definitions, knowledge, and attitudes. J Am Coll Surg. 2005;200:103–10.
10. Bracken-Roche D, Bell E, Karpowicz L, Racine E. Disclosure, consent, and the exercise of patient autonomy in surgical innovation: a systematic content analysis of the conceptual literature. Account Res. 2014;21:331–52.
11. Lantos JD. The "inclusion benefit" in clinical trials. J Pediatr. 1999;134:130–1.
12. Ivy EJ, Lorenc PZ, Aston SJ. Is there a difference? A prospective study comparing lateral and standard SMAS face lifts with extended SMAS and composite rhydectomies. Plast Reconstr Surg. 1996;98:1135–43.
13. Fost N. Ethical dilemmas in medical innovation and research: distinguishing experimentation from practice. Semin Perinatol. 1998;22:223–32.

14. Biffl WL, Spain DA, Reitsma AM, et al. Responsible development and application of surgical innovations: a position statement of the Society of University Surgeons. J Am Coll Surg. 2008;206:1204–9.
15. Lee Char SJ, Hills NK, Lo B, Kirkwood KS. Informed consent for innovative surgery: a survey of patients and surgeons. Surgery. 2013;153:473–80.

16. Semantics and Patient Perceptions of New Technologies

David R. Urbach

The word *technology* has an overwhelmingly positive connotation. People experience new technologies constantly throughout their daily lives, and their own personal experience provides them with a clear notion of the value of the technologies they interact with. For example, people recognize that their newer electronic devices, such as mobile telephones and televisions, represent clear improvements over the devices that were available only a few years ago. Gordon E. Moore, the co-founder of the Intel Corporation, observed in 1965 that the number of transistors in an integrated circuit chip doubles approximately every 2 years. This so-called Moore's Law largely explains the stunning growth of computing power over the past decades, and why computing-based technologies improve so quickly. There is an increasingly prevalent belief that newer technologies are improvements over older technologies. This chapter will explore how the words and language used to describe and characterize new technologies influence patient perceptions about the value of the technology.

New Health Technologies

There are important differences in how products are valued and appraised, depending on whether they are used personally by a consumer, or whether they are used on behalf of a consumer by an agent. An example of a client-agent relationship is a surgeon using a new technology in the care of a patient. A consumer can assess for themselves whether a newer plasma television monitor is better for them than their existing television monitor, and can make an informed decision about whether its cost—both

© Springer International Publishing Switzerland 2016   171
S.C. Stain et al. (eds.), *The SAGES Manual Ethics*
of Surgical Innovation, DOI 10.1007/978-3-319-27663-2_16

economic and noneconomic—justifies its purchase. In the case of tech-nologies used by surgeons in the medical treatment of their patients, consumers are typically not in a position to be able to completely assess the value of the technology themselves and rely on their surgeons to make these judgments. Further, the effectiveness of surgical technologies is not as readily apparent to a user as the effectiveness of consumer products. A person can test drive a new car and get a fairly good idea of how it compares to the car they currently drive. There is no similar opportunity for a patient to "test drive" different technologies or devices that may be used to perform their operation.

There is uncertainty about the effects of health technologies when they are used in the treatment of patients. The body is a complex system, and it is impossible to predict exactly how well a technology will perform in an individual patient. Further, there is often a lack of reliable clinical evidence about the benefits and harms of new technologies. Agencies that regulate health products, such as the US Food and Drug Administration (FDA), generally require high-quality evidence from randomized controlled trials prior to providing a license to market new pharmaceutical agents. However, the standard of clinical evidence for nondrug technologies, such as medical devices, is much weaker. For some low-risk products (such as a new wheel-chair), all that is necessary is an establishment license, demonstrating that a manufacturing facility utilizes appropriate general controls, such as using good manufacturing processes. Many new technologies are approved under the FDA's 510(k) pathway, which requires only that an existing product is substantially equivalent to a licensed product. For example, an endoscope fitted with variations of existing linear or circular surgical staplers might be approved under the FDA's 510(k) pathway on the basis of similarity to existing endoscopes and surgical staplers, even though the clinical effects and risks of the new devices may be quite different [1]. Even when new evidence is required for market approval, this evidence may take the form of engineering or animal studies, or small uncontrolled clinical evaluations in a relatively small number of patients.

Language Used to Describe Health Technology

The problem of technology is further complicated by the importance of the language used to characterize and promote health products. The words used to describe a new technology have a major influence on how the technology is understood. This includes not only how surgeons describe new devices or procedures to patients, but also how manufacturers advertise and market their products, to both surgeons and directly to patients themselves. Advertising relies heavily on latent symbolism in addition to explicit descriptions of a product or service. Product advertisements have both a signifier (the object) and a signified (a concept). The signified has both *denotative* and *connotative* meanings. For example, the denotative meaning of an advertisement for a surgical robot is that it is very precise and minimally invasive. The connotative meaning is that it is a state-of-the-art treatment [2]. Marketing communication claims may be either objective or subjective. Objective claims relate to the measurable attributes of a product or service. Subjective claims evoke emotional or subjective aspects [3]. There is a large body of evidence that suggests that surgeons and patients are influenced by the words used to describe technologies.

Expertise and Acceptability of Technology

Rao and colleagues [4] explored the acceptability of innovative surgical techniques to the general population using the examples of natural orifice transluminal endoscopic surgery (NOTES) and single-port surgery for appendectomy. A questionnaire survey was administered to 736 subjects, including physicians, nurses, and the general public. Subjects were asked "The use of single port laparoscopic and NOTES techniques are relatively new and the safety profile is not fully established. Would you still consider the newer options for your operation without knowing how safe they are?" While 34 % of subjects overall said they would choose one of the newer techniques, there was a significant difference of opinion among subjects according to their clinical background: only 29 % of physicians chose one of the two new techniques, as compared with 35 % for the general population and 49 % for nurses. While some of the divergence of opinion was explained on the basis of sex, this study is noteworthy for how it explains the reluctance of surgeons to themselves undergo new and innovative procedures, despite their willingness to perform them on patients.

Patient Education and Perceptions of Surgical Technology

The relationship between a patient's level of education and information and his or her willingness to undergo a new procedure is complex. On the one hand, more informed or better-educated patients may perceive new technology in a more positive way because of their special knowledge or experience in other dimensions of their lives. On the other hand, they may be more skeptical consumers and not willingly undergo procedures without convincing evidence of its safety and effectiveness. Swanstrom and colleagues [5] surveyed 192 patients about attitudes toward NOTES and laparoscopic surgery for cholecystectomy. 56 % of patients preferred notes over laparoscopic cholecystectomy. Patients with a college education were more likely to choose NOTES than those without a college education. Eighty percent of patients choosing NOTES still would prefer it if it carried slightly greater risk than laparoscopic cholecystectomy, 18 % would still prefer it if the risk was much higher, and 21 % would still prefer it if they were the first person operated on by the surgeon.

Willingness to Pay for New Technology

Schwartzkopf and colleagues [6] surveyed 101 patients undergoing total knee and hip arthroplasty to assess the value they placed on new technology. Eighty percent of subjects responded that they would not be satisfied with a "standard of care" prosthesis, and 86.4 % said they would be willing to pay out of pocket for a prosthesis that was "higher" than the "standard of care." Socioeconomic status, ethnic group, and type of insurance did not affect patients willingness to pay for an implant prosthesis. The authors concluded that patients place value on new technology that they view as an upgrade and would be willing to share in the cost of a prosthesis if it represented a possible upgrade from "standard of care" as they perceive it. Patients prefer having the option to choose an innovative implant with possible advantages, even if the "out of pocket" cost is higher.

Language and Patients' Perceptions of Technology

Dixon and colleagues [7] studied how language influenced patients' decision-making about new surgical technologies, using the case of robot-assisted surgery, which is becoming an increasingly popular method of performing minimally invasive surgery. The evidence on the relative efficacy and safety of robotic surgery is limited, and robot-assisted surgery is significantly more expensive than alternatives including conventional laparoscopic surgery. Therefore, it is likely that the large increase in the number of robot-assisted surgery procedures performed is due to other factors.

One possibility is that advertising and marketing activities influence patient perceptions about technology. The Internet is an increasingly common source of health information, and websites of robotic technology manufacturers often use terms like "innovative" and "state-of-the-art" to describe their products. However, no study had directly assessed the impact of marketing words on patient preference for surgical techniques. The authors of this study sought to determine how these promotional terms influence patient preference for robotic surgery when compared to more neutral language about the value of the technology.

The study surveyed thirty-eight 18- to 75-year-old English-speaking patients attending an ambulatory surgical clinic for an unrelated purpose, to elicit their preference of surgical technique for resection of a localized colon cancer. Each respondent was asked twice to decide between conventional laparoscopic or robot-assisted partial colectomy. In one of the two treatment decisions, robot-assisted surgery was described as a "state-of-the-art, innovative new technology" (the "marketing" frame) and in the other a "promising new technology, which has not been used extensively and with research regarding its safety and effectiveness ongoing" (the "evidence-based" frame).

The median age of study participants was 52 with an approximately equal distribution of sexes. The most commonly reported current state of health was "very good" (34 %), and the majority of subjects had a surgical history (71 %). Under the marketing frame, 20 subjects (52.6 %, 95 % CI 37.2–67.5) chose robot-assisted surgery. Of these subjects, 12 (60 %, 95 % CI 38.7–78.1) switched their choice to conventional laparoscopic surgery under the evidence-based frame. All but one of the 18 subjects who chose conventional laparoscopic surgery in the marketing frame made the same decision under the evidence-based frame. Among the 13 participants who made discordant treatment decisions under opposing frames, robot-assisted surgery was significantly more likely to be chosen under the marketing frame than the evidence-based frame. The likelihood of selecting robot-assisted surgery under the marketing frame and not the evidence-based frame was significantly higher among older participants (odds ratio, 4.8; 95 % confidence interval, 1.1–25.8 for those above the median age [52 years] vs. those below).

The findings suggested that marketing strategies unrelated to the presentation of potential risks and benefits of a surgical technology may influence patient preference. Subjects were more likely to select robot-assisted surgery over conventional laparoscopic surgery when it was described as "innovative" and "state-of-the-art" as compared to when the description included disclosure of the limitations of available evidence. The magnitude of the framing effect was large; 12 of 38 (32 %) selected robot-assisted surgery in the marketing frame and not the evidence-based frame. This effect may be contributing to rising trends in the number of robot-assisted surgery procedures performed.

An explanation for the rising popularity of robot-assisted surgery is the influence of marketing pressures. Objective assessments of the information provided in direct-to-consumer advertising reveal a consistent overstatement of the benefits and understatement of risks not only by manufacturers and distributors of robot-assisted surgery technology, but also by healthcare providers [8]. This is particularly concerning since members of the medical community are in a unique position in that consumers assume the information they provide is unbiased and factually correct.

Direct-to-consumer advertisements promote the novelty of robot-assisted surgery using terms, which include "innovative," "state-of-the-art," or "cutting-edge." These terms may have an important influence on patient preference for new technology. This effect may in part be explained by the conception that the most recently developed treatments represent an accumulation of previous knowledge and must therefore be the best treatments available.

Role of Patient-Physician Interaction

There is evidence that peoples' initial positive perception of novelty in health technology can be tempered by in-depth discussion of the risks and benefits of the procedures. Hey and colleagues [9] studied patient perspectives on single-incision as compared with conventional multiport laparoscopic cholecystectomy. They prospectively studied 133 consecutive patients awaiting elective cholecystectomy. Patients were first shown postoperative images of patients who had undergone both of these procedures and asked about their preference. Subsequently, subjects completed a questionnaire with three components: (1) using published data on the outcomes of cholecystectomy (postoperative pain, cosmetic outcome, recovery time, operative variables), subjects responded to statements about how acceptable each item was for each procedure; (2) participants responded with their preference for each procedure in light of statements about issues related to the introduction of the new technology (technical difficulty for a surgeon, cost); and (3) subjects ranked eight factors—complications, cosmetic result, cost, surgeon experience, operative duration, novelty of the procedure, number of incisions, and postoperative pain—in order of importance with respect to selecting a surgical procedure. Finally, subjects viewed the postoperative images of single-port and conventional multiport cholecystectomy and were again interrogated about their preference.

Initially, 37 % of subjects preferred single-incision laparoscopic cholecystectomy, 27 % had no preference, and 16 % preferred multiport laparoscopic cholecystectomy. After completing the questionnaires, there was a striking change in opinion: only 10 % now preferred single-incision laparoscopic cholecystectomy, 2 % had no preference, and 88 % preferred conventional multiport laparoscopic cholecystectomy. The factors most highly ranked with respect to importance for choosing the procedure were the risk of complications and pain. The least important factor was the novelty of the procedure.

This study highlighted the importance of providing comprehensive information to patients, to ensure that superficial considerations of cosmetic results and novelty do not unduly outweigh clinical benefits, such as risks, benefits, and clinical outcomes.

Summary

There is a large amount of evidence that the language used to describe health technologies has an important influence on how technologies are perceived by patients. Terms that emphasize novelty and innovation are associated with more appealing connotations than terms that emphasize the uncertainty or experimental nature of many new technologies. Patients value new technology and are willing to pay a premium for it. Surgeons appear to be more willing to use new technologies on their patients than they would be to undergo a procedure using new technology themselves. The ability of language to influence patients to undergo new surgical procedures can be moderated by more extensive communication between the surgeon and the patient.

References

1. Maisel WH. Medical device regulation: an introduction for the practicing physician. Ann Intern Med. 2004;140(4):296–302.
2. Umiker-Sebeok DJ. Marketing and semiotics. Berlin: Walter de Gruyter & Co.; 1987.
3. Koc E. Impact of gender in marketing communications: the role of cognitive and affective cues. J Mark Commun. 2002;8(4):257.

4. Rao A, Kynaston J, MacDonald ER, Ahmed I. Patient preferences for surgical techniques: should we invest in new approaches? Surg Endosc. 2010;24:3016–25.
5. Swanstrom LL, Volckmann E, Hungness E, Soper NJ. Patient attitudes and expectations regarding natural orifice transluminal endoscopic surgery. Surg Endosc. 2009; 23:1519–25.
6. Schwartzkopf R, Sagebin FM, Karia R, Koenig KM, Bosco JA, Slover JD. Factors influencing patients' willingness to pay for new technologies in hip and knee implants. J Arthroplasty. 2013;28:390–4.
7. Dixon PR, Grant RC, Urbach DR. The impact of marketing language on patient preference for robot-assisted surgery. Surg Innov. 2015;22(1):15–19.
8. Mirkin JN, Lowrance WT, Feifer AH, Mulhall JP, Eastham JE, Elkin EB. Direct-to-consumer internet promotion of robotic prostatectomy exhibits varying quality of information. Health Aff (Millwood). 2012;31(4):760–9.
9. Hey J, Roberts KJ, Morris-Stiff GJ, Toogood GJ. Patient views through the keyhole: new perspectives on single-incision vs. multiport laparoscopic cholecystectomy. HPB. 2012;14:242–6.

17. Tracking Outcomes of New Technologies

Rizwan Ahmed, Chady Atallah, and Anne O. Lidor

> *Because professionals sometimes do more harm than good when they intervene in the lives of other people, their policies and practices should be informed by rigorous, transparent, up-to-date evaluations*
> *Sir Iain Chambers—Founder of Cochrane Collaboration, 2003, Annals of the American Academy of Political and Social Science*

The collaboration between surgeons and the biomedical industry has resulted in ever evolving series of innovative technologies designed to benefit and improve outcomes among surgical patients. A well-known example of this collaboration was the introduction of laparoscopy. When the first laparoscopic cholecystectomy was done on a human in 1985, there was widespread skepticism from both patients and surgeons. Fast-forward three decades later, the laparoscopic cholecystectomy has become the standard approach for performing a cholecystectomy. This revolutionized the patient's experience of having their gallbladder removed in terms of pain, surgical scars, wound infections, hospitalization, and length of recovery. All in all, the introduction of laparoscopy changed the patient experience for the better. However, currently there are a plethora of new surgical innovations, and the challenge faced by the surgical community is to determine which of these innovations are beneficial or harmful to patients. The objectives of this chapter are: (1) to discuss the ethical concerns of new surgical technology, (2) explore how databases were utilized to improve the outcomes among surgical patients, (3) describe which database resources are currently available, and (4) suggest what components a database should have in order to address new technologies.

© Springer International Publishing Switzerland 2016   179
S.C. Stain et al. (eds.), *The SAGES Manual Ethics*
of Surgical Innovation, DOI 10.1007/978-3-319-27663-2_17

The Ethical Concerns and New Technologies

Based on the evolution of laparoscopic surgery, today's surgical community has a better understanding of the fact that surgical techniques taught to current surgical residents are likely to be outdated in future. While general surgical residents are being trained in laparoscopic and robotic surgery, the advertisement of "scar-less" surgery generated an interest toward Natural Orifice Transluminal Endoscopic Surgery (NOTES). The next generation of surgical devices and new procedures may improve patient care in a way current surgeons cannot fathom. Introduction of new improved surgical devices will happen, and these technologies are bound to change the operative approach and improve the surgical patient experience.

However, there are also ethical concerns. One must keep in mind that most devices are developed by the biomedical and device industry for financial gain. This in turn leads to a potential conflict of interest when a technology is introduced. For industry to be successful, they need to first convince the surgeon that their technology is superior. In order to do so, industry may sponsor research studies. In the era of evidence-based medicine, clinicians are more likely to accept the results of peer-reviewed medical publications. This may be worrisome as a recent Cochrane review concluded that industry-sponsored studies were more likely to report results in favor of the sponsor's product when compared to the results of studies which had no industry sponsorship [1]. Industry also advertises their products directly to patients, encouraging patients to, "ask their doctor about" a particular product. Industry's information can be misleading to a patient who does not understand the gravity of their disease and the intricacies of their operation. Ultimately, the surgeon claims accountability when using a new technology.

As surgeons, in order to provide the optimal surgical care to our patients, our obligation is threefold. First, we are obligated to know which new technology is either beneficial or harmful to our patients. Second, we are obligated to adapt and learn how to use new devices or perform new procedures. Third, it is our responsibility to provide our patients with the most accurate and up-to-date information, devoid of industry's bias, regarding new technologies, and involve patients in the decision-making process toward their own surgical care.

In the past, studying outcomes has been the crux of improving surgical care. One of the first surgical databases was created by Dr. William Halsted at the Johns Hopkins Hospital, Baltimore, Maryland. He began collecting data from patients afflicted with breast cancer that underwent a Halsted mastectomy. As our understanding of imaging and tumor biology improved, American College of Surgeons Oncology Group Z11 trial was conducted and showed that breast conserving management was possible for certain forms of breast cancer [2]. Surgeons transitioned from the Halsted mastectomy to a breast preserving surgery. This is one on the many examples how using databases allowed the surgical community to track outcomes and identify which surgical practices were beneficial or harmful to patients.

Benefits of Tracking Outcome: Cardiac Surgery Experience

The surgical community can learn from historical approaches that improved patient care and apply them to new surgical techniques and medical devices. We describe the evolution of how cardiac surgery improved their performance by developing and utilizing national databases in order to track patient outcomes.

Originally in 1972, the Cardiac Surgery Consultants Committee (CSCC) was established to monitor cardiac surgical care within the Veteran Affairs Health System (VA). They pioneered the use of risk-adjusted analysis to an existing large pool of data collected from cardiac surgery patients who had undergone treatment in the VA system. They then conducted multiple studies and projects using this database to better understand which practices led to better outcomes by giving cardiac surgeons feedback. For instance, one of these studies showed that there was a significant decrease in the risk of postoperative atrial fibrillation among patients who received a pre-operative loading dose of amiodarone and beta-blockade [3].

Following this, in 1989, the Society of Thoracic Surgeons (STS) developed a voluntary nationwide surgeon-driven database for cardiac surgery, which allowed hospitals (other than the VA system) to contribute their data. Similarly, the STS database allowed researchers and institutions to benchmark their outcomes against national averages, thus changing their practices and improving their performance. Edwards et al. reported a landmark study that utilized the STS database and had a significant impact on patient survival. They reported that using internal mammary artery (IMA) as a conduit in coronary artery bypass graft (CABG) decreased the operative mortality from 4.5 to 2 % when compared to the use of venous conduits alone [4]. This study's finding initiated a national and then international shift, and cardiac surgeons began using the IMA when feasible in CABG operations. These experiences from cardiac surgery emphasize the importance of collecting granular data at a national level in order to identify which medical and surgical practices were beneficial or detrimental to patients.

The Creation of National Surgical Databases

Although the existing databases improved outcomes among cardiac surgery patients, there was still a need to address the various other surgical specialties. This led to the creation of more comprehensive surgical databases at a national level. Two such examples are the National Surgical Quality Improvement Program (NSQIP) and the Surgical Care Improvement Program (SCIP).

In the early 1990s, morbidity and mortality rates in VA hospitals were perceived to be higher than national averages. This resulted in the enrollment of 44 VA hospitals in the National VA Surgical Risk Study (NVASRS) that was conducted from 1991 to 1993. This allowed a comparative quality measurement of surgical care in regard to intra-operative and 30-day mortality and morbidity in nine different surgical specialties. As a result of that study, NSQIP was created in 1994 as a database to track and measure outcomes in the VA healthcare system. Data analysis would result in feedback to healthcare providers, in the form of periodic assessments, structured site visits, identification, and dissemination of best practices. A 27 % drop in postoperative mortality and a 43 % drop in morbidity were observed from 1991 to 2006 in participating hospitals [5]. Subsequently, the American College of surgeons (ACS) began enrolling hospitals from the private sector into ACS NSQIP, which has now become the first nationally validated risk-adjusted outcomes-based program to track and analyze data and improve surgical care quality and performance in the USA.

Currently, on a national level, ACS NSQIP provides over 400 hospitals with tools and analyses to improve surgical outcomes. As a result, hospitals can compare themselves to the national average and identify specific areas where quality improvement is needed. Moreover, this large pool of data is utilized for the creation of evidence-based recommendations such as the Best Practice Guidelines (BPGs), which are periodically updated and provided to all participating hospitals. Sharing NSQIP data has therefore proven to improve outcomes related to surgical care. However, the challenge for new technologies is that NSQIP does not provide resources to track new technologies, and thus, we cannot utilize NSQIP to evaluate the safety, effectiveness, and complications of innovative surgical technologies and devices.

In 2003, Centers for Medicare and Medicaid Services (CMS), the largest purchaser of healthcare in the USA, were concerned about the significant morbidity and increasing cost of surgical complications, which led to the creation of SCIP. It consisted of a number of measures aimed at decreasing surgical site infections (SSI), venous thromboembolisms, and postoperative cardiac events. Reporting on these measures was made mandatory, which in turn increased compliance of providers and hospitals and improved surgical outcomes and performances. Reports have shown an 18 % decrease in the odds of developing an SSI, with an actual cumulative decrease of 4 % in SSI [6].

Current Databases and New Technologies

The experiences from NSQIP and SCIP highlight crucial role of national databases in improving surgical outcomes. However, these databases are not modified in a timely fashion to accommodate the pace of new surgical technologies, which in turn leads to a delay in analyzing the outcomes of such advances. We discuss the early challenges of single incision laparoscopic surgery (SILS) and robotic surgery.

The biggest challenge faced when introducing a new technology is to find an appropriate platform to report its outcomes. A poignant example is how SILS was in wide practice before the current procedural terminology (CPT) codes were developed. This forced surgeons to continue using prior CPT codes. As a result, there are no accurate patient records from the early SILS experience, thus preventing the accurate assessment of SILS early complications and long-term outcomes.

There are ethical challenges as well when new technologies have no standardized reporting system. An example of this was inaccuracies and deficiencies in reporting of adverse events in robotics surgery. Specifically, investigators found underreporting of deaths following robotic surgeries. In fact, cases from two electronic databases, LexiNexis and Public Access to Court Electronic Records (PACER), were cross-referenced with the Food and Drug Association (FDA) database. Over a course of 12 years, there were total of 71 peri-operative mortalities among patients that underwent robotic surgery. However, when complications were submitted to the FDA, robotic manufacturers did not report five deaths and inaccurately reported another three mortalities [7].

It is crucial that adverse events related to new medical devices be captured and reported adequately and promptly, in order to assess the device's safety. Currently, manufacturers are required to report device-related complications within 30 days to the FDA. However, providers are not obligated to report those complications, which unveils the problem of a voluntary database with no real oversight or enforcement. Furthermore, the differentiation between device-related adverse outcome and human error is not always evident, and manufacturers have used this argument to avoid accurately reporting complications about new devices to the FDA.

Evidently, surgical societies and governmental institutions have recognized these issues. Significant efforts are currently ongoing to make necessary modifications to the current databases and reporting systems in order to address these concerns.

Ideal Framework and FDA

Realizing the need to improve reporting standards in surgery while addressing practical and methodological challenges, Iain Chalmers, founder of the Cochrane collaboration, with a group of experts in Oxford, England, developed the IDEAL framework. It outlines the process for evaluating new procedures and techniques to allow surgeons to safely and effectively incorporate them into their practice [8]. The components of the IDEAL framework are explained further in Table 17.1. While the IDEAL framework addresses new procedures, it does not address new devices. Developers of the IDEAL framework have suggested that the framework can also be used to assess new technology.

The FDA has taken on the responsibility to assess new technologies related to healthcare since 1971. However, the system that was in place did not meet the challenges of rapidly evolving medical devices. Therefore, following recommendations from the Institute Of Medicine (IOM), the FDA implemented a new device surveillance strategy, which included the creation of the Total Product Life Cycle (TPLC) database. This online transparent directory, easily accessible to the public, included comprehensive records of pre-and postmarket activity for medical devices, as well as manufacturer and user device experience, adverse events, and product recalls.

As part of that same strategy, the FDA held a public workshop in December 2011 entitled "Bridging the IDEAL and TPLC approaches for evidence development for surgical medical devices and procedures,"

Table 17.1. The five stages of the IDEAL framework.

1. *Idea:*
Early after the idea of a new procedure is developed and implemented on a human subject, there should be appropriate online reporting on a searchable registry, including adverse events.
2. *Development:*
Once this new technique has been tried out and as part of the inevitable early stage of rapid modification, there should be clear and comprehensive accounts of when and why techniques are changed, as well as reporting of each patient considered for the procedure sequentially, as opposed to the much less informative and biased case series format of reporting outcomes.
Protocols should be clearly established on an online registry.
3. *Exploration:*
Preliminary prospective cohort studies should be done by surgeons attempting to develop randomized trials together. This usually aims at reducing the uncertainty about the trial population, but it also helps in assessing the surgeons' learning curves as they begin to perform this new procedure, using validated methods such as CUSUM.
4. *Assessment:*
The next stage of development would be assessment of this new technique by randomized controlled trials.
5. *Long-term outcomes:*
Once the technique has been accepted and studied, there needs to be comprehensive registries that should be as complete as possible in terms of data entry, including all adverse events.

aimed at dealing with issues related to evaluation of new surgical devices and tracking of long-term outcomes [9]. Among other recommendations, four actions were proposed to improve postmarket surveillance of medical devices: (1) establish a unique device identification system and incorporate it in the electronic health information system, (2) promote the development of national and international device registries, (3) modernize adverse event reporting and analysis, and (4) develop and use new methods for evidence generation, synthesis, and appraisal.

Tracking Outcomes at a National and an International Level

The development of NOTES and Peroral Endoscopic Myotomy (POEM) is described in further detail elsewhere in this publication. However, the way their outcomes are tracked is interesting and the surgical community can learn for these experiences. A unique aspect of the POEM experience was the globalization of data collection. Data were pooled from 16 expert centers across North America, Asia, and Europe, which allowed surgeons to analyze 841 POEM procedures and provided a snapshot of how practices varied among centers. The different experiences from these centers, including patient selection, technique, and adverse events, were made available for comparative studies and prompted surgeons to comply with what was considered "better practice" to improve their outcomes. That also allowed a global consensus about a new technique that was exponentially growing and thus minimizing the uncertainties that surgeons faced when they first started performing it on patients [10]. However, there is irony in the way POEM is currently in practice. Despite the benefits of tracking outcomes that popularized and made POEM a safe procedure, to date there is no voluntary reporting of POEM. This is concerning as the POEM procedure is being performed by both surgeons and gastroenterologist with no oversight, and we will be unable to ascertain which techniques are most beneficial to patients in the short and long term.

Along the same lines, NOTES, appealing to patients who desired scar-less surgery, began emerging in a few centers; however, specific safety and consensus guidelines were lacking. To address that problem, EURO-NOTES Clinical Registry was established as a voluntary online registry to allow the safe introduction of this new technique to different European countries. The other important feature of that database is that data were recorded in an anonymous way, allowing surgeons to report adverse outcomes more freely and without worry of blame or reprehension. In 2 years, the large pool of data and outcomes made it possible for European surgeons who had access to that registry to safely and effectively perform NOTES in their practice [11].

Proposal for a Perfect Database

Drawing from the previous experiences the surgical community has faced, we should consider the past experiences as lessons to address tracking outcomes of new technologies, after comprehensively evaluating the evolution of current surgical databases and challenges faced when introducing a new technology. In Table 17.2, we list components that a potential database should have in order to address new technologies.

Table 17.2. The components of a database for tracking new technologies.

1. An electronic database that tracks all the information about patient outcomes including clinical information and information related to the surgical procedure

2. A compatible standardized reporting system across all hospitals that allows data linkage with other well-developed databases

3. A device-specific dataset that needs to be defined to measure outcomes to eliminate inaccurate reporting of adverse events in a "free-text" format, with continuous update of the dataset to accommodate all new problems encountered with the device

4. A readily available and affordable system to be used for postmarket surveillance, with the cost shared by health-care providers, industry, and government

5. An anonymous reporting system, to prevent providers concern for reprehension or blame

6. A system allowing patient self-reporting of adverse events

7. An electronic software that allows randomized controlled trials

8. An international and borderless database, with ease of access and sharing of data among different countries

9. A database that preserves patient anonymity and autonomy and allows patient access to a de-identified dataset including risks and benefits of a device

Once the "perfect" database for tracking new medical devices is established, the information gathered and recorded would have to be studied and analyzed periodically, and continuous feedback should be given to individual providers and to institutions. The feedback can be given in different ways, including but not limited to: (1) periodic reports to both providers and manufacturers regarding specific outcomes and adverse events, (2) self-assessment tools and comparative measurements to allow improvements in both technical aspects of a procedure and mechanical features of a device, (3) on-site visits to identify specific procedural and methodological difficulties related to new technologies. The latter would likely require adequate funding to include experts in medicine and in engineering for those visits, hence the need for industry, government, and the surgical societies to share the cost and responsibility.

Sages and New Technology

Moving forward, whenever a new technology is introduced, we need to revisit the fundamental principle of surgery, which is to provide the best care to our patients. The Society of American Gastrointestinal and Endoscopic Surgeons (SAGES) have been at the forefront in celebrating new surgical technologies that improve patient care. However, we should celebrate new advances with caution and use them wisely in order to avoid the scenarios that we have discussed. Our task is to develop a platform for future surgeons and equip them with resources to evaluate new technologies wisely so that they can provide the optimal care to their patients.

Acknowledgments The views expressed in this chapter are the responsibility of the authors alone and do not necessarily reflect the views or policies of SAGES, nor does mention of trade names, commercial products, or organizations imply endorsement by the US Government. The authors of this manuscript have no conflicts of interest to disclose.

References

1. Lundh A, Sismondo S, Lexchin J, Busuioc OA, Bero L. Industry sponsorship and research outcome. Cochrane Database Syst Rev. 2012 Dec 12;12:MR000033. doi:10.1002/14651858.MR000033.pub2.
2. Giuliano AE, Hunt KK, Ballman KV, Beitsch PD, Whitworth PW, Blumencranz PW, Leitch AM, Saha S, McCall LM, Morrow M. Axillary dissection vs no axillary dissection in women with invasive breast cancer and sentinel node metastasis: a randomized clinical trial. JAMA. 2011;305(6):569–75.
3. Halpin LS, Barnett SD, Burton NA. National databases and clinical practice specialist: decreasing postoperative atrial fibrillation following cardiac surgery. Outcomes Manag. 2004;8(1):33–8.
4. Edwards FH, Clark RE, Schwartz M. Impact of internal mammary artery conduits on operative mortality in coronary revascularization. Ann Thorac Surg. 1994;57(1):27–32.
5. Khuri SF, Daley J, Henderson WG. The comparative assessment and improvement of quality of surgical care in the Department of Veterans Affairs. Arch Surg. 2002;137(1):20–7.
6. Munday GS, Deveaux P, Roberts H, Fry DE, Polk HC. Impact of implementation of the Surgical Care Improvement Project and future strategies for improving quality in surgery. Am J Surg. 2014;208(5):835–40.
7. Cooper MA, Ibrahim A, Lyu H, Makary MA. Underreporting of robotic surgery complications. J Healthc Qual. 2013;27.

8. Hirst A, Agha RA, Rosin D, McCulloch P. How can we improve surgical research and innovation? The IDEAL framework for action. Int J Surg. 2013;11(10):1038–42.

9. Transcript for public workshop – bridging the IDEAL and TPLC approaches for evidence development for surgical medical devices and procedures. 2011. Available at http://www.fda.gov/MedicalDevices/NewsEvents/WorkshopsConferences/ucm288553.htm. Accessed 2 Dec 2013.

10. Stavropoulos SN, Modayil RJ, Friedel D, Savides T. The international per oral endoscopic myotomy survey (IPOEMS): a snapshot of the global POEM experience. Surg Endosc. 2013;27(9):3322–38.

11. Arezzo A, Zornig C, Mofid H, Fuchs KH, Breithaupt W, Noguera J, Kaehler G, Magdeburg R, Perretta S, Dallemagne B, Marescaux J, Copaescu C, Graur F, Szasz A, Forgione A, Pugliese R, Buess G, Bhattacharjee HK, Navarra G, Godina M, Shishin K, Morino M. The EURO-NOTES clinical registry for natural orifice transluminal endoscopic surgery: a 2-year activity report. Surg Endosc. 2013;27(9):3073–84.

18. Balancing the Surgeon's Responsibility to Individuals and Society

Bruce D. White and Luke C. Gelinas

Cutting-edge and progressive physicians and surgeons innovate [1].[1] Indeed, innovation may at times rise to the level of a moral obligation, one that springs from the doctor's ethical and legal responsibility to practice medicine and surgery competently. Ethical physicians must be competent practitioners, which means they must be alert to the ever-changing aspects of medicine and incorporate newer and better methods and technologies into patient care whenever appropriate. As Pellegrino emphasized: "[A doctor] binds himself to competence as a moral obligation" and "places the well-being of those he presumes to help above his own personal gain" [2]. Competent physicians are watchful, observant, and open-minded, and they continuously re-evaluate how better to provide quality care in its many aspects, from washing one's hands (as suggested by Semmelweis in the 1850s) [3], to ligating a patent ductus arteriosus (as did Gross in 1938) [4], to considering complementary and alternative interventions today [5]. Many therapeutic innovations—not just improvisations which appear prudent, but thoughtful, considered, and indeed groundbreaking improvements in treatments—derive from the innovative practices of competent physicians and may not always be proven or established by prospective double-blinded, randomized controlled trials, or some other similar irrefutable evidentiary standard. However, this does not mean innovations are not evidence-based and grounded in accepted medical practices.

---

[1]*Innovate (v.)* means "to introduce something new." Anne H. Soukhanov, exec ed (1992). *The American Heritage Dictionary of the English Language.* Boston: Houghton Mifflin Company, p. 931.

© Springer International Publishing Switzerland 2016
S.C. Stain et al. (eds.), *The SAGES Manual Ethics of Surgical Innovation*, DOI 10.1007/978-3-319-27663-2_18

Unfortunately, and perhaps too often, when physicians and surgeons think about innovating to improve patient care or delivery processes, they worry about liabilities, including medical malpractice, and other ethical and legal concerns. Of course, this happens with the full knowledge that many nonprofit institutions and organizations exist with the acknowledged purpose of promoting quality improvement and innovation in medical and surgical practice [6]. But still, physicians are rightfully anxious about the ethical and legal implications of trying a new technique or a new drug (or an approved drug for an unapproved use) because of possible charges of unprofessional or tortious conduct, even if unfounded or unmeritorious. Allegations of improper practice and liability are relatively infrequent but unmistakable reminders to surgeons of their responsibilities to patients and the community.

Physicians and surgeons should take heart though in recalling that innovation is traditionally an inherent part of good medical practice. Most patients and medical care plans and providers understand that good doctors continually look for ways to improve care and technique. To be sure, innovation should not take place in a vacuum, by physicians acting in isolation from their peers in the wider medical community. Instead, competent physicians innovate within the evidentiary framework provided by the current state of their profession, modifying practices to reflect current peer recommendations and suggestions about best practices [7].

Two "Innovation" Cases: 1767 and 2013

Somewhat surprisingly, the ethical and legal responsibilities with regard to innovative approaches and therapies have not changed radically over the years. What has changed has been the available technology, which has progressed and advanced unabated, making more and more complex innovations possible [8]. There are, undoubtedly, proportionately more medical malpractice cases in the USA now than just 50 years ago, but the ethical and legal obligations have remained the same and are arguably applied more even-handedly in practice today than ever before [9]. Just two cases—centuries apart—might help illustrate the relatively uniform way in which the law has dealt with bad outcomes associated with ill-advised innovative surgeries over time.

One of the first reported medical malpractice opinions in the English law reports dealt with an innovative or "experimental" surgery case [10]. The patient—a Mr. Slater—had broken two bones in one of his legs. A surgeon and an apothecary initially attended him. (The written opinion does not give the first surgeon's name; John Latham was the apothecary involved early on. Both of these professionals testified at the subsequent trial.) Nine weeks after the injury, the patient's two broken leg bones had healed sufficiently for the patient to "go home" and walk with crutches. There is some question in the judges' written opinion about whether or not the leg had healed correctly or aligned well, but it was clear that a calculus had formed. During the relatively long recovery, a second "eminent" surgeon from St. Bartholomew's Hospital and another apothecary—Messrs. Baker and Stapleton—began seeing the patient as well. These two providers saw Slater at least three times during his convalescence. The patient's daughter testified at trial that Apothecary Stapleton had been called to change the bandage but declined to do so without the assistance of Surgeon Baker. When Baker and Stapleton saw Slater the third time, there was some "alteration" in their clinical approach. Doctor Baker had an "instrument" or "machine" he wanted to "put on" the patient in an "operation of extension." It is unclear from the opinion as to why the operation was considered necessary. However, during the "operation," it was certain that Baker and Stapleton rebroke the patient's leg. The judges wrote that the patient did not agree or consent to the "operation." The court's decision in the case turned on whether the plaintiff gave informed consent to the innovative surgery. In a *per curium* opinion, the court held that Baker and Stapleton had acted rashly and "unskilfully" [sic] and gave judgment to the plaintiff Slater. The judges labeled the "operation" an "experiment." Of course, the treatment plan did deviate from the standard of care as established by the patient's first surgeon-apothecary team, and one may unquestionably describe the Baker-Stapleton intervention as innovative.

If one were to fast forward about 250 years to the present, it would remain obvious that physicians and surgeons have continued to innovate in caring for patients in spite of any risks associated with accusations of unethical, unprofessional, or substandard conduct in care delivery. For example, *The Sacramento Bee*—in a series of newspaper articles in early 2013—reported on an "innovative" neurosurgery intervention that caused a scandal at the University of California (UC) Davis Medical Center (UCDMC) [11]. Two neurosurgeons understood the dismal short- and long-term survival statistics for patients with brain cancer, specifically glioblastomas. After very lengthy reflection and professional discussions with others, they came to believe that if the immune systems of glioblastoma patients could be sufficiently stimulated, their survival might be improved. It was a reasonable corollary to the understanding that disease and stress dramatically compromise the immune system. Moreover, this belief was grounded in anecdotal reports and a sketchy literature review that appeared to show that patients with concurrent bacterial infections while undergoing treatment for glioblastomas fared somewhat better than patients who did not have concurrent infections. The UC Davis neurosurgeons and several other physicians came to believe that these concurrent infections somehow stimulated the patients' immune systems and thus helped fight the cancer. The neurosurgeons felt that one way to test this hypothesis was to implant relatively benign or minimally harmful bacteria into the surgical site after the greatest bulk of the glioblastoma had been resected from the patient's brain. At UC Davis, when they initially raised this possibility with the director of the Institutional Review Board (IRB), they were allegedly told that IRB approval would not be necessary for a very small number of patients since the procedure was "innovative" and thus exempt from IRB oversight [12].

The whole story as it played out is far more complicated, involving notably, what appeared to be, questionable motives on the part of the surgeons in design and execution. But even this rough sketch of events shows the linkage between innovation and experimentation and how existing extensive organizational oversight infrastructure exists for the former, but not necessarily the latter. By early 2013, after the death of three glioblastoma patients who had consented to the innovative procedure, both neurosurgeons had been roundly condemned for violating university policies. Both eventually left the medical center under clouds. As an immediate consequence, the university promulgated an "Innovative Care Policy" to govern similar situations in the future [13].

Unfortunately, it is all too easy for some to say that an innovative intervention was "experimental" as happened in these two cases centuries apart. With bad outcomes, plaintiffs' attorneys and prosecutors will undoubtedly use the experiment label to incite or inflame juries, judges, and medical board members and the public in an attempt to show that doctors failed to act as reasonably prudent practitioners in providing optimal care to patients. It may take determined effort on the part of physicians and their defenders and supporters to help decision makers and regulators better understand the nuances and subtleties when innovative interventions are offered as compared with clinical research and other similar concepts.

Definitions

Like Justice Potter Stewart in trying to define obscenity (who wrote "I know it when I see it") [14], some surgeons might say that it is hard to define *innovation* and distinguish it from improvisation and experimentation,[2] or even novel[3] operations performed infrequently. The terms may be hard to demarcate, but these are words used in everyday practice, making it useful to attempt to characterize them as precisely as possible. As such, it is valuable to review how innovation is different from improvisation and experimentation, as well as the different standards for informed consent in each type of case. This will also provide opportunity to reflect on the extent of the ethical responsibility to innovate and how best to accomplish this as one practices good medicine. Table 18.1 provides key markers for distinguishing or differentiating the terms and ideas and their application in practice.

Perhaps the best way to attempt to define "innovative surgery" is to compare and contrast it with other akin concepts. Innovative surgery can be located on a continuum between clearly accepted, conventional, or mainstream approaches, procedures, and techniques on the one end, and experimental surgery on the other end [15]. The spectrum is organized primarily around the degree to which different types of surgical interventions are accepted and practiced in the surgical community. The more widely accepted and commonly practiced a type of surgical intervention is, the closer it will fall to the conventional or mainstream end of the spectrum; the "newer" or less widely accepted and less commonly practiced, the closer to the experimental end. Because the risks of a surgical intervention can be expected to correlate reliably with the degree to which that intervention is accepted and practiced by the medical community—with better-accepted and more widely used practices generally being less riskier than less well-accepted ones—the spectrum is also characterized by increasing risk, and so increasing safeguards and standards for informed consent, as we move from widely accepted surgery toward novel and experimental surgery.

---

[2] *Experiment* (*v.*) means "to test under controlled conditions that is made to demonstrate a known truth, examine the validity of a hypothesis, or determine the efficacy of something previously untried." Anne H. Soukhanov, exec ed (1992). *The American Heritage Dictionary of the English Language.* Boston: Houghton Mifflin Company, p. 645.

[3] *Novel* (*adj.*) means "strikingly new, unusual, or different." Anne H. Soukhanov, exec ed (1992). *The American Heritage Dictionary of the English Language.* Boston: Houghton Mifflin Company, p. 1239.

Table 18.1. Improvisation, innovation, experimentation, and novel infrequently performed procedures.

Intervention	Use foreseeable?	Use intended prior to procedure?	Timing of decision to intervene (intentional)?	Preintervention informed consent obtained?	IRB approval?	Example?
Necessary improvisation	Perhaps	No	In the moment, use unanticipated; not-premeditated	No; but the law may authorize such interventions in an emergency (an extension of the "doctrine of necessity") so long as the surgeon was not in fact responsible for the "emergency" through negligence	No	A surgeon encounters a problem or a complication during a procedure that requires an imaginative response (perhaps an emergency, perhaps not)
Elective improvisation	Yes	No	In the moment, use seen as a possibility but not planned; not-premeditated	No	No	A surgeon has insight into a different approach during a procedure but intervention was not anticipated nor necessary
Innovation	Yes	Yes; thoughtfully, reflectively	Planned; premeditated	Yes, structured but individualized	No	Ligation of a patent ductus arteriosus (Gross 1938)
Research or "Experiment"	Yes	Yes; quite deliberately, systematically	Planned; premeditated	Yes, formally structured and uniform	Yes	A surgeon participates in a randomized controlled trial
Novel, infrequently performed procedure or operation	Yes	Yes; quite deliberately, systematically	Planned, premeditated	Yes, structured and individualized	No	Hemicorporectomy; separation of conjoined twins

To begin on the widely accepted end of the spectrum, it is important to recognize that there can be variation within the standard of care itself. Historically, medical tort law has recognized this fact in the "locality rule," which establishes different standards for malpractice depending on the medical customs and practices specific to different geographical locales. The locality rule doctrine is based on the assumption that the standard of care that it is reasonable for patients to expect quite literally changes from place to place. Although technology and ease of information sharing are poised to make the locality doctrine a thing of the past (as of 2007, 29 states and the District of Columbia had accepted a "national standard," with 21 states retaining a local-based standard), variation within the conventional standard of care persists [16]. Indeed different approaches to the same medical problem will equally count as standard of care whenever there is equipoise or genuine uncertainty in the medical community at large over which one of multiple existing therapies is most effective—not an uncommon state of affairs.

It is also important to see that even the most widely accepted surgical procedures remain susceptible to unforeseen obstacles and challenges, calling for flexibility, and time-sensitive decision-making on the part of practitioners. Surgeons will always be faced with the task of tailoring decisions, in an immediate way as situations unfold, to the complexities of particular patients and circumstances. That is, surgeons must often *improvise* to be successful. One can distinguish two types of improvisation: the first may be termed *necessary improvisation* and the second, *elective improvisation*.

Both forms of improvisation, necessary and elective arise in response to the particularities of specific patients and circumstances and involve *unplanned* alterations to a surgical course of action. The key difference is that necessary improvisation involves circumstances that *require* an emergent or nonemergent change of plan in the moment to optimize surgery success, while elective improvisation is not required in the same way. For example, a necessary improvisation might involve a surgeon changing her planned method or manner of excision of a mass to avoid excessive risk—for example, to accommodate an unanticipated cluster of blood vessels in order to safely remove the mass. Elective improvisation, by contrast, is not required in this same way. An elective improvisation is an unplanned course of action undertaken in the moment that in the practitioner's eyes constitutes an *improvement* over his or her planned technique, while not being strictly required for the success of the surgery. For example, a surgeon stitching up an incision may decide that one way of placing sutures is better and more conducive to healing than another way of placing them, even if both techniques would ultimately result in good healing.

Both necessary and elective improvisations are likely to be relatively common aspects of surgical practice. Moreover, because both types of improvisation are unplanned, there is no opportunity to obtain extensive consent for them prior to surgery, if such consent would be required at all. In the case of necessary improvisation, commonly accepted ethical and legal standards, such as the "doctrine of necessity," will typically justify surgeons proceeding with the unplanned improvisation, at least when a better outcome or the patient's safety is at issue. It is a more interesting question under what conditions elective improvisation is justified and (assuming it is at least sometimes justified) *why* it is justified.

Approaching the main target, innovative surgery resembles improvisational surgery in that both involve unique or modified surgical techniques that are not conventional or mainstream practice. But whereas the improvisational surgeon adopts nonconventional techniques in response to contingencies as they arise in the moment during surgery, the innovative surgeon reflectively *plans* to employ new techniques as part of the surgical procedure before surgery begins. Moreover, to distinguish innovative surgery from clinical research, the intention to employ nonconventional surgical techniques must be based on a judgment that the nonconventional technique in question will benefit *this particular patient*. Innovative surgery is the thoughtful and intended use of new and nonconventional surgical techniques, toward the end of benefitting the patients undergoing the operation.

Consider, for example, the history of the Blalock-Taussig shunt [17]. In 1943—after the idea was rejected by very experienced and skilled pediatric surgeons—cardiologist Helen B. Taussig approached Alfred Blalock and Vivien Thomas at their Johns Hopkins lab with the possibility of a shunt that would mimic the physiologic function of a patent ductus arteriosus and improve outcomes in infants with cyanotic heart defects [18]. Blalock and Thomas were intrigued by the idea and set about refining the procedure in dogs, after which Blalock attempted the surgery on human infants, with great success. Blalock would go on to perform the procedure on scores on infants, significantly improving their quality of life. The history of the Blalock-Taussig shunt provides what we take to be a paradigm case of successful "innovative surgery," with surgeons intentionally and thoughtfully employing novel techniques and available technological means to improve the care of individual patients.

There is one important thing to note about the account of innovative surgery sketched here: the relation between innovative surgery and clinical research. Innovative surgery differs from clinical (or "experimental") research primarily by virtue of an intention in their aims and purpose. Whereas clinical research aims at generalizable conclusions, putting aside personalized care of patients for the prospect of valuable medical knowledge, innovative surgery, as commonly understood, is always undertaken as part of a personalized plan of care for individual patients. To count as innovative surgery, rather than research, a nonconventional surgical procedure or technique must be pursued primarily *because* it is likely to benefit a particular patient, not because it will let us derive generalizable knowledge. The personalized aim of innovative surgery is reflected in the fact that, unlike clinical research, surgeons who innovate do not employ a control group or test two interventions against each other. It is also, one might argue, what lies behind the fact that innovative surgery does not require IRB approval to be morally or legally acceptable and defensible.

The UC Davis Medical Center instituted a policy on innovative care as part of a plan of correction submitted to the California Department of Public Health investigation into the neurosurgery case discussed earlier. The relevant sections support our account of the distinction between innovation and research and may help shed additional light on the concept [13]:

> *Innovative care*—is the application of a therapy, device, or medication to a patient in a manner that departs in a significant way from standard or accepted medical practice in order to enhance the well-being of a specific patient. The sole purpose of innovative care is to benefit the patient, not to collect data to support a hypothesis or theory. Innovative care includes any use of an unapproved drug, biologic, or device that is subject to Food and Drug Administration (FDA) expanded access approval. Innovative care also includes unusual or entirely novel off-label uses of FDA approved drugs, biologics, or devices, but does not include common off-label use. For the purposes of this policy, innovative care and compassionate care are synonymous.[4]

Another very good example of an innovative and experimental procedure that has become more conventional or mainstream over the last

---

[4] It may be curious that the policy drafters at UCDMC would equate innovative care and compassionate care. Others would certainly disagree. Compassionate care may be used as an exception to carve out a deviation from nonconventional treatment because it is in the patient's best interest to do so, but compassionate care to many implies a life-limiting or life-threatening situation that is not always essential for one to invoke an innovative care approach also to be used in the patient's best interest.

several years is the serial transverse enteroplasty (STEP) procedure for pediatric short gut syndrome. The originating surgical team theorized a possible solution and attempted it first in young pigs [19]. It was then attempted successfully in a 2-year boy born with gastroschisis and midgut volvulus that left him total parenteral nutrition (TPN) dependent [20]. Probably as a best practice, the team involved the hospital's Clinical Investigation Committee to help oversee the first clinical case; more than likely this mechanism was used rather than the hospital's IRB since the intervention was an "innovation" exempt from IRB approval. Now surgical teams at leading children's hospitals around the country offer the intervention as a conventional standard of care treatment [21].

Finally, one should also distinguish improvised, innovative, and experimental surgeries from novel, infrequently performed operations, such as a hemicorporectomy and the separation of conjoined twins. Hemicorporectomies are performed rarely, perhaps most often by surgeons who would have never attempted the operations before. But it would be hard to believe that a team of surgeons (probably including general surgeons, orthopedic surgeons, vascular surgeons, and trauma surgeons, and more broadly, anesthesiologists and critical care intensivists and cardiologists and pulmonologists as well as others) would ever undertake such an exhaustive operation without thorough reflection, planning, and even technical practice. Infrequency does not necessarily imply that the operation is innovative; if the procedure is reported widely and well described, it is not new. Of course, for infrequently performed operations, the informed consent process would most likely be as extensive as that required for experimental operations or clinical research projects to assure that the patient completely understood the associated risks and benefits.

Over time—as one might expect—the innovations will be adopted or rejected by prudent and skilled practitioners. The innovations will thus convert to conventional or mainstream interventions or remain as options when clinical circumstances arise for novel but infrequently used treatments, or may become more widely available later as technological advances permit. Figure 18.1 illustrates this conversion or relabeling. Also Fig. 18.1 shows how the conventional and novel are nonexperimental, separate from clinical research. The nonexperimental interventions over time are employed in patient's best interests, whereas the experimental are employed to test hypotheses or advance generalizable knowledge. However, one should recall though that the novel,

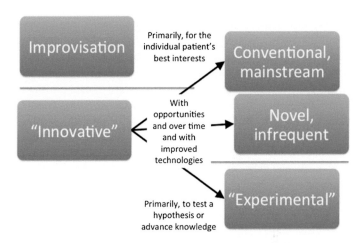

Fig. 18.1. *The transformation or conversion of "Innovative" interventions over time.* With application and adoption or rejection over time, innovative treatments are reclassified because they are incorporated into conventional practice or offered infrequently because of specific clinical circumstances or because surgeon investigators develop research protocols to test hypotheses to advance generalizable knowledge in the field.

infrequently employed interventions are still more similar to the experimental than the conventional and mainstream in the level of information that should be shared with patients or legally authorized representatives in obtaining authentic informed consent to proceed.

Risks, Outcomes, and Foreseeability

All surgeries carry risk. Unfortunately, some of the risks associated with innovative, experimental, and novel surgeries will not be foreseeable. For those risks that are foreseeable, the surgical team should be able to deal with them in ethically and legally appropriate ways as part of the informed consent process [22]. However, liability may turn less on foreseeable risk than on bad outcomes [23]. A patient or a patient's legally authorized representative that is pleased with the surgical outcomes will see no harm or injury and will have no reason to sue for damages or complain to an institution or state medical board [24]. But unforeseen bad outcomes are an inherent part of surgical practice and can be expected statistically. And no matter how much care is taken *ex ante*, bad outcomes are likely to lead to allegations of unethical, unprofessional, and substandard conduct, that is, to charges of malpractice or misconduct. When unforeseen bad outcomes do eventuate, one should not forget that innovative surgeries can be standard of care practice; and the best defense in a malpractice suit will be that the surgeon met the standard of care [25]. At the same time, since the ultimate outcomes of most complicated and extensive surgeries are unpredictable, it would be unwise for surgeons to suggest anything close to a guaranteed or definitive end result, and to be candid and up-front about the possibility of bad unforeseen results [26, 27].

Moreover, the motives and intentions of surgeons in these situations matter. If the surgery is innovative, the more it appears that the surgeon was motivated to act in the patient's best interests, and the patient's best interests alone, the better. This motive will typically allow one to infer that the reason the surgeon employed an innovative technique—the surgeon's *intent* in doing so—was to improve the patient's condition. This is likely to mitigate emotions of blame and anger that patients and families, as well as representatives of the legal system, might be inclined to feel in cases where innovative surgery results in unforeseen bad outcomes. By contrast, when the motive to benefit patients is mixed or clouded—as it was with the UC Davis neurosurgeons' case—it will be much more tempting to conclude that the surgery was experimental: designed primarily to test a hypothesis, rather than provide top-tier personalized care. In the UC Davis case, the neurosurgeons' premeditated actions clearly led reviewers to believe that the doctors had conflicts of interests and were motivated by self-interest in addition to the patients' best interests.[5] Motives of self-interest on the part of surgeons will make cases of innovative surgery with bad outcomes more difficult to defend before the law.

[5] From one of the surgeon's own well-circulated accounts of the incident, he had conversation with a National Institutes of Health pediatric oncologist and ethicist about the project when soliciting IRB support; he worked energetically to identify the better bacterial culture option to implant and settled on a "locally-grown" product; he investigated the idea of commercially marketing the bacterial material; after treating two patients he elected to ignore IRB advice to seek an investigational new drug application (IND) before treating subsequent patients; and he was aware that other similarly situated investigators were operating under the authority of government-funded research protocols rather than any color of "innovative" intervention. [12]

Surgical Innovation and Informed Consent

Appropriately documented informed consent or informed refusal is widely acknowledged to be a foundational norm of both the law and medical ethics [25]. The moral and legal obligation for caregivers to obtain informed consent stems most basically from the duty to respect patient autonomy and the rights of patients to control their own bodily space [28, 29]. Traditionally, informed consent requires patients to comprehend several pieces of information. It requires patients to have a basic understanding of what is involved in the procedure being offered, its likely risks and benefits, as well as the risks and benefits of alternative procedures (including foregoing procedures altogether). It is also widely agreed that informed consent requires *voluntary* assent on the part of the patient. While some cases of innovative surgery raise questions about whether the voluntariness requirement is or can be met—namely, those in which the innovation proposed is the only possible or last available way to treat an urgent medical problem—these issues arise in other cases and are not specific to innovative surgery. On the other hand, innovative surgery does raise a distinctive set of questions about the understanding requirements of informed consent.

One may start by assuming that the amount of information a patient or legally authorized representative needs to make a decision varies with the degree of risk involved in the procedure. Figure 18.2 attempts to graphically illustrate this feature of informed consent. Major elective surgery, for example, carries more stringent disclosure requirements than routine or minor surgery, and life-saving surgery carries more stringent disclosure requirements than major elective surgery. Keeping this in mind, we will also assume that for consent to innovative surgery to be genuinely or authentically informed, patients must at a minimum meet the usual understanding requirements for informed consent, that is, those operative in cases of noninnovative, conventional surgery (and generally): they must have a basic grasp of what is involved in the procedure, its risk and benefits (described at the appropriate level of detail, depending on the seriousness of the surgery), and the risks and benefits of alternative procedures. This suggests that adding innovation into the informed consent or informed refusal equation shifts the curve depicted in Fig. 18.2 to the left, calling for more information to be shared than for standard treatment without the innovative component.

Three beliefs follow directly from these related assumptions. First, whenever innovative surgery carries *different risks* than alternatives,

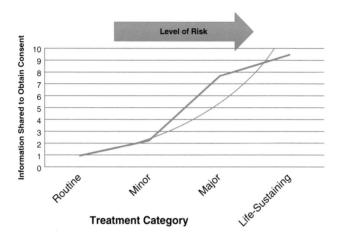

Fig. 18.2. *Level of information to be shared to obtain valid informed consent.*
The vertical axis displays the scaled amount of information to be offered and
how more—rather than less—information should be offered as the risks increase
along the horizontal axis. One might think that by introducing innovation into
the equation that the curve will shift to the left with all treatment categories:
requiring more information to be shared with the patient if the risks increase.

surgeons are obligated to disclose these differences in risk, at least when
the surgery is neither routine nor very minor. For example, if single-port
laparoscopic cholecystectomy (which we will assume currently counts
as "innovative") carries different risks than more conventional (multiport) laparoscopic cholecystectomy, surgeons are obligated to disclose
the differences between them. Note that the idea here is not (or not
merely) that surgeons should disclose that one procedure might be
riskier than another. The reason persons may expect disclosure of *different types* of risks, rather than relative riskiness *per se*, is that different
patients may weight potential risks differently, depending on the badness
different patients attach to different outcomes and physical states. The
surgeon may and arguably should assist the patient in reflecting on how
best to balance the risks involved with different procedures, depending
on the ill consequences the patient assigns to possible outcomes. But the
determination of overall risk-differential between different possible surgeries will often depend on the patient's values and require discussion
and dialogue with her.

Second, and perhaps no less important, whenever innovative surgery
carries different likely *benefits* than alternatives, surgeons should also

disclose the different benefits. Because well-informed choice between two treatment alternatives requires knowledge of their different possible benefits, no less than knowledge of their risks, similar points made earlier with regard to risk apply here.

While these points about the need to disclose the different risks and benefits of alternative interventions seem to us undeniable, it is an open and interesting question how often surgeons practicing innovative surgery will themselves have insight into the real risks and benefits associated with innovative procedures. Surgeons willing to use innovative procedures over more accepted ones presumably do so because they think the innovative option is in some way preferable to the accepted one: that its risk-benefit ratio is better for the patient. Of course, this does not always turn out to be true. Extracranial-intracranial arterial bypass for ischemic stroke, for example, was eventually found to correlate with increased risk of stroke, and knee arthroscopy for osteoarthritis was likewise eventually deemed ineffective [30–32]. What makes things difficult, with respect to adequately informing recipients of innovative therapies, is the possibility that the benefit the caregiver perceives will turn out to be merely illusory, as well as the possibility of unforeseen risks. These dangers appear to be an essential part of novel therapies as well.

So far as promoting adequately informed consent, perhaps the safest route is for surgeons to be up-front and candid about the possibility that the benefits they perceive are just that—perceived, not yet proven—as well as about the possibility of unforeseen risks. As noted, even the most common and well-accepted surgeries may not turn out to benefit patients and may have unforeseen risks. Surgeons must use prudent clinical judgment to discern whether the prospect of illusionary benefits and unforeseen risks involved with innovative surgery is greater than that involved with more accepted ones. When it is, they should disclose this to patients.

Regarding the third and final point related to informed consent with innovative surgery: if, as standard informed consent doctrine holds, patients must have a basic comprehension about what is involved in a procedure to give informed consent, they must have a view on how the innovative procedure differs, medically speaking, from its alternatives. They must have a hold on what it is about the innovative procedure that distinguishes it from alternatives, such as (for example) that the gall bladder will be removed using only one incision (single-port cholecystectomy) rather than three to four incisions (multiport cholecystectomy). The pressing question here is whether, in addition to basic knowledge of the differences, patients must also be informed *that these differences constitute an innovation* or nonconventional technique for them to be well informed. Should surgeons who propose innovative treatments alert patients to the novel and not quite yet established nature of these procedures?

Several empirical factors may offer insight into this question. First, when theorizing about applicable standards of disclosure for innovative surgery, surgeons can look to their surgical professional societies and associations. While many surgical professional organizations do not go into detail specifying what should be disclosed to recipients of innovative surgeries, the Society of University Surgeons is a notable exception [29]. Its position is that surgeons should disclose the innovative nature and aspects of procedures and that "any omission of such discussion arguably involves deception and violates patient autonomy-based rights to submit to care" [33].

A second source of insight is the actual views and practices of surgeons. A 2002 study by Reitsma and Moreno suggests that most practicing surgeons do in fact inform their patients of the innovative nature of proposed treatments, even if this is not mentioned in the consent form [34]. Perhaps more revealingly, a recent study found that the majority of surgeons think that the innovative nature of procedures *should* be disclosed, with 51 % of surgeons ($n = 85$) saying that disclosure of the new or innovative aspects of a procedure is essential for informed consent in standard surgery, 53 % of surgeons saying that it is essential for informed consent in laparoscopic surgery, and 65 % saying it is essential for informed consent in robotic surgery [30].

Finally, there is the witness of patients themselves. The same survey found comparable support for disclosure of innovation among patients, with 57 % of patients saying that disclosure of the new or innovative aspects of a procedure is essential for informed consent in standard surgery, 62 % saying it is essential for informed consent in laparoscopic surgery, and 63 % saying it is essential for informed consent in laparoscopic surgery [30].

From a normative perspective, it can be argued that any duty to disclose the innovative nature of a procedure is a function of the different or additional risks (if any) that arise from its being new or innovative. If there are situations where a procedure's new or innovative aspects do not carry additional or different risks compared to more accepted alternatives, it is plausible that surgeons are not obligated to disclose its innovative nature. However, since in many cases novel procedures will carry additional and different types of risks, the empirical considerations noted—which support the conclusion that, in the eyes of both patients and surgeons, surgeons are often obligated to disclose the novel status of innovative surgical procedures—seem to point in a morally defensible direction.

Conclusion

While there are real dangers involved with surgical innovation, calling for vigilance in safeguarding patient well-being and autonomy, it is important not to overplay the dangers of innovation, or underplay its benefits. One only needs to consider the history of surgical innovation to appreciate this point [35]. That history suggests that physicians should—to the degree possible—consider, suggest, and provide insightful, studied, and convincing innovative treatments that are peer-acknowledged—accepted, or—reviewed, while taking care to balance their obligation to respect patient autonomy and benefit their patients.

To achieve this balance, it is essential for innovative practitioners to be thoroughly embedded in, and engaged with, peers in the medical community. Because careful physicians are by definition reasonably prudent, they will not act outside a range of acceptable treatment options. Ethically sound innovation must have some basis in theory or peer-acknowledged practice; defensible innovation must be evidence-based, even with the evidence may be more suggestive rather than definitive. Table 18.2 offers several practical pointers for practitioners thinking about employing an innovative intervention in practice.

Table 18.2. Practical pointers for practitioners considering using an "Innovation".

A surgeon who plans or offers an innovative operation, procedure, or technique to a patient might ultimately balance responsibilities to individuals and society better by:

   Consulting with more—rather than fewer—colleagues and peers about concepts and ideas

   Discussing the possibility of innovative surgery with care facility executives and operating room personnel sooner, rather than later

   Sharing more—rather than less—information with the patient about the rationale, and risks and benefits, and use available oversight mechanisms to assure transparency and voluntariness avoidance of conflicts of interests

   Anticipating a worse—rather than a better—outcome, and weighing the risks and benefits in light of this possibility

   Documenting more—rather than less—about the entire idea, decision-making process, planning, and risks and benefits, possible results, and anticipated outcomes

Innovations spring from creative minds through brilliant flashes of inspiration in moments when someone is imagining new possibilities in tackling an old or anticipated problem. But ingenuity alone is not enough, there must be technical wherewithal coupled with the new idea to give the innovation wings. And even then, a careful physician should test hypotheses and application with learned and experienced colleagues who are best suited to challenge the vision and inventiveness. This is the very philosophy undergirding peer review. Peer review has its foundation in the self-regulation of professionals with similar skills sets and competencies. Typically peer review methods—such as those employed in publishing scholarly papers, obtaining grant or foundation support, or in evaluating candidates for academic promotion—are used among experts in a unique discipline or field to provide quality assurance, credibility, and help enhance performance, because other more objective standards are less available. Peer review has long-standing traditions in medicine; it is the best measure available in many situations. New treatments—many unproven—do not spring up overnight. In the exploratory phase, there is no clear line that readily separates the proven from the unproven. Often continual revisions are necessary as innovations evolve for the better [36, 37]. Moreover, regardless of outcomes—whether good or bad, or if innovations meet or fail to meet expectations—ethical physicians are obligated to use suitable means to pass relevant information along to other caregivers, even when the data are potentially embarrassing personally or professionally [38]. Openness and transparency about which treatments are effective or beneficial adds to scientific knowledge and leads to helpful change and better patient care.

References

1. White BD, Gelinas LC, Shelton WN. In particular circumstances attempting unproven interventions is obligatory. Am J Bioeth. 2015;15(4):53–5.
2. Langer E. Edmund D. Pellegrino, prominent bioethicist, dies at 92. The Washington Post. June 19, 2013. http://www.washingtonpost.com/local/obituaries/edmund-d-pellegrino-preiminent-bioethicist-dies-aat-92/2013/06/19/34a3e97a-d82f-11e2-9d14-895344c13c30_s. Accessed 5 Jan 2015.
3. Best M, Neuhauser D. Ignaz Semmelweis and the birth of infection control. BMJ Saf Qual Health Care. 2004;13(3):233–4.
4. Mormile R, Quadrini I, Squarcia U. Milestones in pediatric cardiology: making possible the impossible. Clin Cardiol. 2013;36(2):74–6.

5. National Center on Complementary and Alternative Medicine. National Center on Complementary and Alternative Medicine. 2014. http://www.nccam.nih.gov. Accessed 6 Jan 2015.
6. Institute for Healthcare Improvement. Institute for Healthcare Improvement. March 13, 2015. www.ihi.org. Accessed 13 Mar 2015.
7. Pellegrino ED, Thomasma DC. For the patient's good: the restoration of beneficence in health care. New York: Oxford University Press; 1988.
8. Toulmin S. Technological progress and social policy: the broader significance of medical mishaps. In: Mark S, Stephen T, Zimring FE, Schaffner KF, eds. Medical innovation and bad outcomes: legal, social, and ethical responses. Ann Arbor: Health Administration Press; 1987.
9. Richards RJ. How we got where we are: a look at informed consent in Colorado – past, present, and future. North Ill University Law Rev. 2005;26(1):69–99.
10. *Slater v. Baker and Stapleton.* (English Reports, 1767).
11. Lundstrom M. Impact, Ethics of Surgery Slammed. The Sacramento Bee. February 11, 2013. http://www.sacbee.com/news/investigations/article2576577.html. Accessed 16 Mar 2015.
12. Muizelaar JP. Statement of J. Paul Muizelaar, MD, PhD, in Reply to Investigative Report. The Sacramento Bee. April 22, 2013. http://www.sacbee.com/incoming/article2556180.ece/BINARY/Dr.%20J.%20Paul%20Muizelaar%20statement. Accessed 16 Mar 2015.
13. California Health and Human Services Agency Department of Health. Statement of Deficencies and Plan of Correction: University of California Davis Medical Center. California Department of Public Health. June 12, 2013. http://www.cdpa.gov/certlic/facilities/Documents/2567UCDavisMedCtr-1K5X11-SacramentoCounty.pdf. Accessed 16 Mar 2015.
14. *Jacobellis v. Ohio.* (United States Supreme Court, 1964).
15. Johnson J, Rogers W. Innovative surgery: the ethical challenges. J Med Ethics. 2012;38(1):9–12.
16. Lewis MH, Gohagan JK, Merenstein DJ. The locality rule and the physician's dilemma: local medical practices vs. the national standard of care. JAMA. 2007;297(23):2633–7.
17. Blalock A, Taussig HB. The surgical treatment of malformations of the heart in which there is pulmonary stenosis or pulmonary atresia. JAMA. 1945;128(3):189–92.
18. Freedom RM, Lock J, Bricker JT. Pediatric cardiology and cardiovascular surgery: 1950–2000. Circulation. 2000;102(Supplement 4):IV-58–68.
19. Kim HB, Fauza D, Oh JT, Nurko S, Jaksic T. Serial transverse enteroplasty (STEP): a novel bowel lengthening procedure. J Pediatr Surg. 2003;38(3):425–9.
20. Kim HB, Lee PW, Garza P, Duggan C, Fauza D, Jaksic T. Serial transverse enteroplasty for short bowel syndrome: a case report. J Pediatr Surg. 2003;38(6):881–5.
21. Boston Children's Hospital. International STEP Data Registry. 2015. https://apps.childrenshospital.org/clinical/step. Accessed 29 Mar 2015.
22. Fins JJ. Surgical innovation and ethical dilemmas: precautions and proximity. Cleve Clin J Med. 2008;75 Suppl 6:S7–12.

23. Epstein RA, Zimring FE. Legal liability for medical innovation. In: Siegler M, Toulmin S, Schaffner KF, eds. Medical innovation and bad outcomes: legal, social, and ethical responses. Ann Arbor: Health Administration Press; 1987. p. 162–83.
24. Mastroianni AC. Liability, regulation, and policy in surgical innovation: the cutting edge of research and therapy. Health Matrix. 2006;16(2):351–442.
25. Annas GJ. Standard of care: the law of American bioethics. New York: Oxford University Press; 1993.
26. Thomas R. Lacey's spring woman loses battle with cervical cancer. Decatur Daily. July 31, 2009. http://decaturdaily.com/news/local/lacey-s-spring-woman-loses-battle-with-cervical-cancer/article_e809812edb78-5c38-baad-591d16bdbd80.html. Accessed 17 Mar 2015.
27. Grondahl P. Despite operation to cut her in half, angel laughs on. www.timesunion.com. October 21, 2011. http://www.timesunion.com/local/article/Despite-operation-to-cut-her-in-half-Angel-2227298.php. Accessed 17 Mar 2015.
28. Miles SH. The hippocratic oath and the ethics of medicine. Oxford: Oxford University Press; 2004.
29. Annas GJ. The rights of patients. New York: New York University Press (An American Civil Liberties Union Handbook); 2004.
30. Lee Char SJ, Hills NK, Lo B, Kirkwood KS. Informed consent for innovative surgery: a survey of patients and surgeons. Surgery. 2013;153(4):473–80.
31. The EC/IC Bypass Study Group. Failure of the extracranial-intracranial arterial bypass to reduce the risk of ischemic stroke – results of an international randomized trial. N Engl J Med. 1985;313(19):1191–200.
32. Moseley JB, et al. A controlled trial of arthroscopic surgery for osteoarthritis of the knee. N Engl J Med. 2002;347(2):81–8.
33. Biffl WL, et al. Responsible development and application of surgical innovations: a position statement of the society of university surgeons. J Am Coll Surg. 2008;206(6):1204–9.
34. Reitsma AM, Moreno JD. Ethical regulations for innovative surgery: the last frontier? J Am Coll Surg. 2002;194(6):792–801.
35. Bunker JP, Hinkley D, McDermott WV. Surgical innovation and its evaluation. Science. 1978;200:937–41.
36. Centers for Disease Control and Prevention [CDC]. Centers for Disease Control and Prevention. Post-Treatment Lyme Disease Syndrome. August 11, 2014. http://www.cdc.gov/lyme/postLDS/. Accessed 3 Jan 2015.
37. Centers for Disease Control and Prevention [CDC]. Interim U.S. guidance for monitoring and movement of persons with potential Ebola virus exposure. Centers for Disease Control. December 24, 2014. http://www.cdc.gov/vhf/ebola/exposure/monitoring-and-movement-of-persons-with-exposure.html. Accessed 3 Jan 2015.
38. Jena AB, Prasad V, Goldman DP, Romley J. Mortality and treatment patterns among patients hospitalized with acute cardiovascular conditions during dates of national cardiology meetings. JAMA Inter Med (American Medical Associaton), December 2014.

Further Reading

Chang RW, et al. Serial transverse enteroplasty enhances intestinal function in a model of short gut syndrome. Ann Surg. 2006;243(2):223–8.

Office for Human Research Protections, Department of Health and Human Services. Letter from Lisa R. Buchanan, Compliance Oversight Coordinator, to Richard B. Marchase, Vice President for Research and Economic Development, Univeristy of Alabama at Birmingham. Office of Human Research Protection, Department of Health and Human Services. March 7, 2013. http://www.hhs.gov/ohrp/detrm_letrs/YR13/mar13a.pdf. Accessed 17 Mar 2015.

Sacks CA, Warren CE. Foreseeable risks? Informed consent for studies within the standard of care. N Engl J Med. 2015;372(4):306–7.

SUPPORT Study Group of the Eunice Kennedy Shriver NICHD Neonatal Research Network. Target ranges of oxygen saturation in extremely preterm infants. N Engl J Med. 2010;362(21):1959–69.

19. Paying for New Technology: Insurance Company Perspective

Richard Dal Col and Donna Stewart

The rise in health insurance premiums over the past several years has caused the health care industry to redouble efforts to contain costs and maintain affordability. A major factor leading to escalating costs has been the rapid development and dissemination of new technology into the medical marketplace. In order to understand the payer's perspective with regard to paying for new technology, it is essential to understand the relationship between evolution of new technology and health care costs. As described by Rettig, this relationship is a balance between the nation's commitment to health care cost containment and what appears to be the greater commitment to innovation in medicine [1]. He describes five mechanisms of action by which medical innovation (new technology) affects the cost of health care:

1. Major advances create a clinical ability to treat previously untreatable conditions by some long-term maintenance therapy.
2. Secondary diseases within previously untreatable terminal diseases are discovered and major and incremental advances occur in response. Additionally, indications for treatment expand over time, steadily increasing the patient population to which the treatment is applied.
3. Major advances create a clinical ability to treat previously untreatable acute conditions.
4. Incremental improvements in existing capabilities, which are often quality-enhancing, may be cost-increasing and are strongly influenced by coverage and reimbursement decisions.
5. Clinical progress, either by major advances or by the cumulative effect of incremental improvements, extend the scope of medicine to conditions once regarded beyond its boundaries [1].

Rettig concludes it is in the interests of all parties to the medical innovation enterprise to search for ways to accommodate the two

© Springer International Publishing Switzerland 2016
S.C. Stain et al. (eds.), *The SAGES Manual Ethics of Surgical Innovation*, DOI 10.1007/978-3-319-27663-2_19

objectives of ensuring clinical benefit to patients within a given resource constraint and maintaining a continuing flow of highly valued innovations [1]. Health insurance is a method by which members may pool resources and have access to many evolving technologies that on an individual basis may be beyond their financial abilities [2]. As pointed out by the Kaiser Family Foundation, "The presence of health insurance provides some assurance to researchers and medical suppliers that patients will have the resources to pay for new medical products, thus encouraging research and development. At the same time, the promise of better health through improvements in medicine may increase the demand for health insurance by consumers looking for ways to assure access to the type of medical care that they want" [2].

Through adoption of the Institute for Health Care Improvement (IHI) Triple Aim principles (improved health, improved experience of care, cost containment) and commitment to a health value strategy, CDPHP attempts to balance fiduciary responsibility to members while supporting the continuing emergence of innovative technologies in health care. The CDPHP process in assessing new technologies and new applications of existing technologies for inclusion in a benefit plan is a rigorous one, utilizing evidence-based scientific and medical literature as well as determinations from regulatory bodies. In addition, and in keeping with the CDPHP health value strategy, cost containment is balanced with providing support of medical innovation to ensure members have equitable access to safe and effective care.

CDPHP is a physician-founded, member-focused, and community-based not-for-profit health plan that provides services to more than 450,000 members in 24 counties throughout New York and employs over 1000 personnel. The CDPHP Board of Directors, as well as dedicated medical affairs committees (Quality Management, Utilization Management, Pharmacy and Therapeutics, Credentialing, Member Grievance), are composed predominantly of practicing physicians. CDPHP holds National Committee for Quality Assurance (NCQA) Excellent Health Plan Accreditation and was ranked #1 in New York State in 2014 for its commercial and Medicare lines of business. CDPHP sets an annual budget goal of surplus operating income at approximately 2 % with the remainder of the premium dollar divided between hospital costs (31 %), physician costs (24 %), ancillary costs (7 %), administration (12 %), and taxes and fees (8 %).

The CDPHP process for evaluating evolving and currently existing technology is conducted with a focus on triple aim goals and health value strategy and is intended as a means to ensure access to high quality, safe, efficacious, and cost-effective health care. Technology assessment is performed as an ongoing process of monitoring available scientific literature to identify, evaluate, and define the role of new technologies as medically necessary, experimental/investigational, or cosmetic. The technology review process is applied to both the development of new medical policies and the updating of existing policies. The role of the CDPHP Technology Assessment Team (TAT), which consists of medical directors, registered nurses, and additional appointees as needed, is to permit judicious allocation of resources by providing coverage for medically necessary, cost-effective services that reflect current scientific data and accepted standards of clinical practice.

The CDPHP technology review process occurs in five distinct stages and is initiated by an internal request from within the company, from an external source, such as a network provider or hospital, or from landscape review of emerging technologies by the medical policy analyst.

The first stage of the technology review process involves comprehensive research of the proposed technology by a dedicated medical policy analyst. The determination as to whether a technology is safe and/or efficacious is based upon scientific evidence demonstrated in published clinical research. CDPHP considers prospective, randomized, and controlled clinical trials the gold standard of scientific evidence, but recognizes this level of evidence may not be available to guide treatment decisions for all patients with serious disease. CDPHP utilizes the following public and private sources of information in assessing health technologies to establish coverage determinations.

(A) *Professional medical specialty societies and associations guidelines and/or position statements* (e.g., American Medical Association (AMA), American Psychiatric Association (APA), American College of Gynecology (ACOG), American College of Cardiology (ACC))
(B) *Peer-reviewed clinical and scientific literature*

   (a) The Cochrane Library (Evidence for Healthcare Decision Making). Cochrane Library contains a wealth of information regarding diseases, diagnostics, and therapies. The library is a collection of six databases containing high-quality independent evidence that can be accessed and used to make evidence-based health care decisions.[3].
   (b) PubMed Clinical Queries. PubMed allows visitors to search and view studies regarding therapies, diagnoses, and prognoses. PubMed is provided as a free service of the US National Library of Medicine (NLM) allowing access to Medline and NLM databases [4].

(C) *Technology Assessment Entities*

    (a) Hayes, Inc. Hayes technology assessments provide evidence-based assessments of health care technology and critical appraisals of published evidence with a goal of facilitating evidence-based decisions to improve quality and cost-effectiveness of health care [5].

    (b) Center for Clinical Effectiveness (CCE), previously the Blue Cross and Blue Shield Association's Technology Evaluation Center (TEC). CCE provides scientific opinions to health care decision makers provided solely for informational purposes. CCE produces three clinical Resources, The Medical Policy Reference Manual (MPRM), Specialty Pharmacy Reports, and TEC assessments [6].

    (c) Institute for Clinical and Economic review (ICER). ICER is a nonprofit organization whose stated aim is to create a more effective, efficient, and just health care system through collaborative efforts that move scientific evidence into action. ICER's mission is to lead innovation in comparative effectiveness research through methods that integrate consideration of clinical benefit and economic value. ICER does this through two core programs, its original program, the New England Comparative Effectiveness Public Advisory Council (CEPAC) and the California Technology Assessment Forum (CTAF) [7].

    (d) ECRI (formerly the Emergency Care Research Institute). An independent nonprofit health services research agency and a collaborating center of the World Health Organization (WHO). It is designated as an Evidence-Based Practice Center (EPC) by the Agency for Healthcare Research and Quality [8].

    (e) Up-to-Date. This evidence-based clinical decision support resource is authored and peer-reviewed exclusively by physicians recognized as experts in their fields [9].

(D) *Government Agencies*

    (a) US Food and Drug Administration (FDA). The FDA's center for Devices and Radiologic Health (CDRH) offers medical device news, recalls, public health notifications, and guidance documents [10].

    (b) Centers for Medicare and Medicaid Services Council on Technology and Innovation (CTI). The Council on Technology and Innovation oversees coordination of coverage and exchange of information regarding new technologies, procedures, devices, and drug therapies within the Centers for Medicare and Medicaid Services and among other entities [11].

(c) Agency for Healthcare Research and Quality (AHRQ). AHRQ is the lead Federal Agency charged with improving the quality, safety, efficiency, and effectiveness of health care for all Americans. As one of 12 agencies within the Department of Health and Human Services, AHRQ supports health services research that will improve the quality of health care and promote evidence-based decision-making. All AHRQ research is published and available publicly [12].

(d) National Institutes of Health (NIH). This part of the US Department of Health and Human Services serves as the national research agency [13].

(e) New York State Department of Health relating to regulatory compliance.

(E) *Expert opinions from CDPHP board certified network providers and/or recommendations from a CDPHP physician workgroup.*

The second stage in the review process includes an initial review of the completed research by an appropriate medical director, and a recommendation made as to whether the technology requires a formal review by the CDPHP Technology Assessment Team. At this time, and at the discretion of the medical director, expert opinions from participating board certified physicians may be obtained or a workgroup of physicians may be convened when additional expertise is needed regarding a newly emerging medical technology.

Rendering of a coverage determination by the CDPHP technology assessment team constitutes the third step in the review process. CDPHP utilizes all of the five criteria outlined below to reach decisions regarding eligibility for coverage of new or existing technologies and/or procedures. In doing so, CDPHP ensures all benefit coverage decisions reflect current scientific data and medical knowledge and are consistent with current, accepted standards of care. The final determination as to whether the technology meets criteria and is proven safe and/or efficacious is based upon the professional assessment of supporting evidence by the technology assessment team. In addition, a CDPHP medical director may conduct an assessment of a technology for a case-specific review, utilizing the same criteria outlined below and sources of evidence referenced above.

(A) The technology must have final approval from government regulatory bodies. This criterion applies to drugs, biological products, devices, diagnostic technologies, and any other product or procedure that must have final approval to market from the Food and Drug Administration or any other governmental body with authority to regulate the technology.

(B) The scientific evidence must permit conclusions concerning the effect of the technology on health outcomes. The evidence should consist of high-quality scientific studies published in peer-reviewed journals and should demonstrate that the technology can measure or alter the physiological changes related to a disease, injury, illness, or condition. In addition, there should be evidence based on established scientific evidence that the use of this service affects health outcomes.

(C) The technology must improve the net health outcome. The technology's beneficial effects on health outcomes must outweigh any harmful effects on net health outcomes.

(D) The technology must be as beneficial as any established alternatives. The technology should improve the net health outcome as much as, or more than, established standard alternative therapies.

(E) The technology is not cosmetic in nature and is required for reasons other than for the convenience of a member or provider.

The fourth stage in the review process involves outcome decisions by the technology assessment team which may include development of a new policy or revision to an existing policy to address a future covered benefit or to address noncoverage of a reviewed new technology. The CDPHP medical technology assessment team is responsible for determining the need for an external resource coordination policy, while the Pharmacy and Therapeutics Team is responsible for determining the need for a pharmacy policy. In developing policies relating to health technologies, such as medical, behavior health and surgical procedures, pharmaceuticals, diagnostic and screening tests, alternative therapies, and medical devices, CDPHP considers several decision variables including, but not limited to, safety and efficacy, experimental status vs. standard of care, high risk, high volume, issues of controversy, medical appropriateness, regulatory requirements, consistency with CDPHP preventive health and clinical practice guidelines, and cost-effectiveness. All draft policies are presented to the policy committee for review and approval. In addition, draft policies developed to address a new technology or controversial service, or revisions made to an existing policy, may be sent out to clinicians in the CDPHP network for their expert critique and review. The policy committee is a multidisciplinary team consisting of representation from the CDPHP departments of benefit configuration, application management, finance, government programs, internal operations, medical affairs, network and contracting, pharmacy services, business development, special investigation unit, and resource coordination. It is supported by provider consultants in medicine and behavioral health, and workgroups as needed, to lend clinical expertise to the review activities. After approval by the policy committee, the formal draft is presented to the utilization management committee or the pharmacy and therapeutics committee for review and approval. These committees consist of practicing community physicians and pharmacists, appointed by the CDPHP Board of Directors, who represent a cross-section of primary care physicians and specialists from the CDPHP network. Minutes from these respective committees are reported to the quality management committee and board of directors for final approval.

The final stage in the technology review process involves communication to the source of the original request and/or provider network of the new coverage determination and/or policy changes (Fig. 19.1). Updates to resource coordination and pharmacy policies are distributed every other month via mailings and are made available through the CDPHP secure physician interface at www.cdphp.com. Individual policy mailings are performed upon provider or member request.

Recently, CDPHP amended its technology review process to allow for an expedited coverage determination of a new technology. This process would apply only if the technology is believed to be of great benefit to a specific population of patients, or if the given technology is new to the region, and there is a physician or institutional champion who is advocating for its acceptance and early adoption. At the discretion of the medical affairs division, CDPHP will allow the sponsoring physician or institution to directly present a given technology to the medical director team, along with participation of the CEO and senior leadership. The decision to do so is based upon the following factors: the denial process is expensive and cumbersome; there may be unnecessary delay in delivery of the new technology to members; there may be undue burden on physicians trying to advocate for their patients while waiting for coverage determinations to keep pace; and lastly, physicians and institutions could be placed in disadvantaged competitive positions if the process is too lengthy.

In summary, CDPHP utilizes a systematic approach to ensure timely review of emerging technologies and new applications to existing technologies, incorporating principles of the triple aim and health value

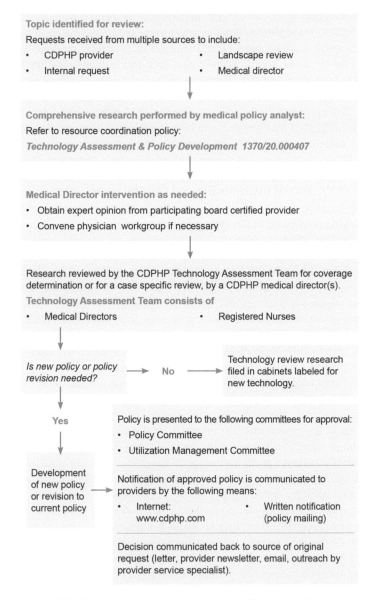

Fig. 19.1. CDPHP new technology review process (Courtesy of Capital District Physicians' Health Plan, Inc.).

strategy. In doing so, CDPHP attempts to balance fiduciary responsibility to members while supporting the continuing emergence of innovative technologies in health care. In response to the cumbersome approval process for a new technology, CDPHP has amended its review process to expedite coverage determinations for a promising or life-altering technology. CDPHP continues to balance cost containment with providing support of medical innovation to ensure members have equitable access to safe and effective care.

References

1. Rettig RA. Medical innovation duels cost containment. Health Aff. 1994;13(3):7–27 (Online). Available at http://content.healthaffairs.org/content/13/3/7. Accessed 15 Jan 2015.
2. Kaiser Family Foundattion 2007. Snapshots: How changes in medical technology affect health care costs (Online). Available at http://kff.org/health-costs/issue-brief/snapshots-how-changes-in-medical-technology-affect/. Accessed 15 Jan 2015.
3. The Cochrane Library. Available at http://www.thecochranelibrary.com/view/0/index.html. Accessed 15 Jan 2015.
4. PubMed. Available at https://www.ncbi.nlm.nih.gov/pubmed. Accessed 15 Jan 2015.
5. Hayes. Available at http://www.hayesinc.com/hayes/. Accessed 15 Jan 2015.
6. Center for Clinical Effectiveness (CCE), previously the Blue Cross and Blue Shield Association's Technology Evaluation Center (TEC). Available at http://www.bcbs.com/blueresources/tec/. Accessed 15 Jan 2015.
7. Institute for Clinical and Economic Review. Available at http://www.icer-review.org/. Accessed 15 Jan 2015.
8. ECRI Institute. Available at https://www.ecri.org/Pages/default.aspx. Accessed 15 Jan 2015.
9. UptoDate. Available at http://www.uptodate.com/home. Accessed 15 Jan 2015.
10. U.S. Food and Drug Administration. Available at http://www.fda.gov/. Accessed 15 Jan 2015.
11. CMS.gov. Centers for Medicare and Medicaid Services. Available at https://cms.gov/Medicare/Coverage/CouncilonTechInnov/index.html. Accessed 15 Jan 2015.
12. Agency for Healthcare Research and Quality (Online). Available at http://www.ahrq.gov/. Accessed 15 Jan 2015.
13. National Institutes of Health. Available at http://nih.gov/. Accessed 15 Jan 2015.

20. Evolving Responsibility for SAGES-TAVAC

Crystal M. Krause and Dmitry Oleynikov

Currently, there are no concise federal regulations regarding innovative surgical procedures or the use of new technology and devices in surgery. A nonbiased method is needed to introduce new technology to surgeons. The Council of Medical Specialty Societies (CMSS) has defined a code for medical society interactions with companies in order to maintain high ethical standards [1]. The main purpose of this code is to maintain objectivity and to decrease conflicts of interest. Societies' interaction with companies may include receiving charitable contributions, applying for grants in support of program activities, and conducting business. The purpose of the code is to guide societies in the development of policies and procedures that safeguard the independence of their programs, policies, and advocacy positions. The CMSS code provides clinical practice guidelines, medical technology assessments, and other clinical practice opinions in order for societies to ethically develop and publish measures or standards for quality or other types of performance [1]. These guidelines were utilized in the development of the Technology and Value Assessment Committee (TAVAC).

In 2012, the Society of American Gastrointestinal and Endoscopic Surgeons (SAGES) established TAVAC in order to provide ethical guidance regarding the use of new procedures and technologies [2]. SAGES has published a number of guidelines for gastrointestinal and endoscopic surgery [3]. The aim of the TAVAC, as well as the responsibility of SAGES, is to help evaluate devices and technology that have been recently approved by the United States Food and Drug Administration (FDA) for safety, efficacy, and to the assess the value that these new technologies bring to patients. To ensure that this process is not biased, TAVAC review panel members are carefully selected

© Springer International Publishing Switzerland 2016
S.C. Stain et al. (eds.), *The SAGES Manual Ethics
of Surgical Innovation*, DOI 10.1007/978-3-319-27663-2_20

so as to not have real or perceived bias, and full disclosure is always required. Conflict of interest is therefore managed by SAGES with the help of peer review.

The Technology and Value Assessment Committee (TAVAC)

The TAVAC was formed to evaluate and make evidence-based recommendations regarding the adoption and use of new and existing technology. Over time, TAVAC may be utilized for guidelines in the use of the new technologies as these technologies become more widely adopted.

TAVAC considers new devices and technologies which are approved for sale in the United States by the FDA. Any SAGES member can request that TAVAC review a particular device or technology. After a preliminary review, the technology undergoes a more detailed assessment and is given one of three possible categorical designations (Table 20.1). Each category requires different levels of evidence to support the end-product of the assessment. That is, a Technology Alert would be for a very new product or device, whereas a Safety and Effectiveness Assessment would be given for a product or device that had been approved for some time and clinical use data would be available for comparison. There are several different processes for FDA approval, and as a result of this, strong clinical data are available more quickly for some devices than others. For example, devices that are cleared through a premarket approval process may have sufficient data available from which to make a determination regarding safety, efficacy, or even a value assessment. On the other hand, the 510 k-approval process may generate very little new clinical data, whereby a Technology Alert may be all that is appropriate.

Table 20.1. TAVAC technology assessment designations.

Assessment designation	Description
Technology alert	Technology or devices that have been recently FDA approved and do not have clinical use data
Safety and effectiveness assessment	Assessment of currently available data to determine if technology meets criteria for safety and effectiveness
Value assessment	Assessment of the value of the technology to practice (V = Quality/Cost)

TAVAC Assessment Designations (AD)

Technology Alert Assessment

A Technology Alert is appropriate for any device recently approved by the FDA where there is insufficient data from which to make any further determination. This would most commonly occur with devices approved through the 510 k process. The 510 k process allows for FDA approval based on a predicate device, where the new device is sufficiently similar to an existing device so as to not require phase I or phase II clinical data before approval. For devices approved in this process, the Technology Alert would detail the intended purpose of the device, summarize the claims by the manufacturer, and speak to the areas where this technology is deemed to be potentially useful once further clinical studies are available. The Technology Alert Assessments conclude with a statement that additional clinical studies are needed before further evaluation can be performed.

Safety and Efficacy Assessment

A Safety and Efficacy Assessment is appropriate for devices that have been recently approved by FDA and where sufficient data are available to make a determination of safety and efficacy. This would typically involve a device that went through the premarket approval process in order to achieve FDA approval. With the premarket approval process, there is usually a requirement of more clinical data than is required in the 510 k-approval process. This additional clinical data may be sufficient to allow SAGES-TAVAC to determine the device to be safe and effective for the intended use. While the FDA has also made such a determination, FDA approval alone often does not convince patients or insurers of the devices safety and efficacy. This usually is due to a limited number of credible and unbiased experts presenting the data to the FDA Advisory Panel. A SAGES-TAVAC assessment of the safety and effectiveness of a device brings added value to the process, possibly enhancing the transfer of new technology into the hands of medical professionals and increasing utilization in patients.

Value Assessment

Assessment of the value of newly proposed technology is appropriate for any readily used medical device, especially given the influence that the cost of devices and procedures has on the utilization in the patient. Value in health care is defined as a ratio of quality over cost; a high-value procedure would be one of high-quality and low-cost. A value assessment of technology would be appropriate for any device which is readily available for use, but where its role and value in the care of patients remains unclear. The value assessment would be very useful for physicians to balance their responsibility as an individual patient advocate and also their responsibility to society in the stewardship of finite health care resources [2].

The TAVAC Assessment Process

Depending on the initial assessment designation (AD), SAGES-TAVAC follows a specific process in order to make an unbiased assessment of the technology. The end-product of the evaluation is a statement or publication through the SAGES website [4].

Each TAVAC AD requires a different process for review and final determination. TAVAC amasses a roster of SAGES members who have expertise related to different technologies. Broad categories of expertise in clinical areas or specific technology are developed (e.g., gastroesophageal reflux disease, colorectal disease, endomechanical devices, electrosurgery). SAGES members who are interested in participating in the TAVAC will be solicited to perform assessments within their area of expertise. Anyone participating in an assessment for TAVAC is required to undergo a review for potential conflicts of interest. This aspect of the assessment process is critically important. Incidences of inappropriate or mismanaged financial relationships between physicians, industry, and even professional medical associations contribute to the dissemination of biased information, possibly confounding data and contribute to the erosion of public trust [5, 6].

When a request to TAVAC for an assessment is received, the Chair or his/her designee performs a preliminary review to determine the appropriate AD. The requestor can specify a category for assessment, but the final decision as to the actual assessment performed is the decision of the TAVAC Chair.

To determine the proper AD, a panel of experts is convened to review all available data. Again, critical to the panel composition is transparency regarding any potential conflict of interest. Whenever possible, expert panel members without potential conflict of interests are utilized. A panel of five members is convened for each assessment, and a Panel Chair is identified. Administrative personnel are assigned to each assessment project and assist the panel Chair with acquiring needed data, organizing panel discussions, meetings and calls, and preparing the final document to be published on the SAGES website. One panel member is expected to have experience and/or expertise in surgical administration or healthcare management related to managing supplies or equipment for an operating room. This person is typically a department or division chair, surgeon-in-chief, or part of a hospital's administrative leadership team. At least one panel member has experience and/or expertise in outcomes research and analysis, including performing cost analysis. Data focused on outcomes and cost are reviewed and summarized, and particular attention will be paid to current standards of care and costs from which to be able to compare the value of the new device or technology. The end-product of the panel's work will vary depending on the assessment designation. For example, in cases where a value assessment designation is given, the end-product of the assessment will be a manuscript published in Surgical Endoscopy. This manuscript would follow an expedited review and publication timeline. The results of the individual device or technology panel's assessment will be reviewed by the TAVAC for final approval, and ultimately the final result of the assessment will be approved by the SAGES Board of Governors.

Conclusion

The development of medical devices and technologies by engineers cannot and does not occur independently of physicians. This device-industry-physician relationship is essential to the advancement of procedural medicine [2]. With the development of new devices and products, education and training on the particular device or technology is necessary in order to safely introduce the product into clinical practice. The maintenance of ethically sound relationships between professional medical associations, such as SAGES, and the industries developing new devices and technologies is essential to the safe dissemination of new information and devices to the practicing physician. Surgical societies function to fill the gap that currently exists between FDA approval of a medical device and marketing by a device manufacturer. The SAGES-TAVAC, with the help of expert surgeons, evaluates new technology and devices and gives guidance as to the proper place and value for these new technologies. This type of guidance is particularly valuable because it is free of commercial bias and potential conflict of interest is managed through peer review. Maintaining an ethical and fair review of new medical devices and technology is essential. One study has shown that the citation of a medical device in a journal has an impact on the marketing and adoption of the device, potentially increasing the product's market value by up to 3 % [7]. The value of TAVAC is not only in the release of nonbiased information on new devices and technologies to physicians, but the resulting assessments from the TAVAC can be utilized by entities that regulate physician practice, including state hospitals and insurance payers. Due to the lag-time between availability of a device and in the absence of long-term clinical studies, these TAVAC assessments are useful in that they provide additional information about technologies that are unavailable in the published literature. The assessments help to show the utility of a new device or technology and its potential role in today's constantly evolving healthcare.

References

1. Council of Medical Specialty Societies. Code for interaction with companies. 2011. http://www.cmss.org/codeforinteractions.aspx.
2. Strong VE, Forde KA, MacFadyen BV, Mellinger JD, Crookes PF, Sillin LF, Shadduck PP. Ethical considerations regarding the implementation of new technologies and techniques in surgery. Surg Endosc. 2014;28:2272–6. doi:10.1007/s00464-014-3644-1.
3. SAGES Resource Guide. 2015. http://www.sages.org/about/resources/.
4. SAGES Clinical/Practice/Training Guidelines, Statements & Standards of Practice. 2015. http://www.sages.org/publications/guidelines/.
5. Healy WL, Peterson RN. Department of Justice investigation of orthopaedic industry. J Bone Joint Surg Am. 2009;91:1791–805. doi:10.2106/JBJS.I.00096.
6. Schafer K, AAD questions sunscreen seal program. 2008. http://www.cosmeticsandtoiletries.com/regulatory/uvfilters/16745326.html. Cosmetics & Toiletries Science Applied.
7. Chatterji AK, Fabrizio KR, Mitchell W, Schulman KA. Physician-industry cooperation in the medical device industry. Health Aff (Millwood). 2008;27:1532–43. doi:10.1377/hlthaff.27.6.1532.

21. Evolving Responsibility for SAGES: New Technology Guideline

Robert D. Fanelli

The Society of American Gastrointestinal and Endoscopic Surgeons (SAGES) has earned the well-deserved reputation as the premier membership organization for general surgeons worldwide. Its origin and focus remain centered on technological innovation through the clinical platforms of flexible endoscopy and minimally invasive surgery. In its role as a professional society formed to bring structure to the myriad disruptive technologies that have shaped modern surgery and endoscopy throughout the last 35 years, SAGES has great responsibility for guiding its membership and has established the Guidelines Committee to advise membership in issues related to training, novel procedures, and clinical practice. In 2014, SAGES published guidelines related to the ethical introduction of new techniques and technologies into clinical practice [1]. This chapter is based in part on the guideline creation process, on a presentation given at the 2014 Annual SAGES Meeting, and on the SAGES guideline itself.

The Ethical Perspective

An ethical approach to patient treatment is a principle central to the clinical practice of surgery. The solutions to patient problems and health care challenges rarely are black and white, and an ethical foundation allows clinicians to make decisions from an informed and considerate perspective so that entire populations are treated with equipoise. A discussion of the origins of medical ethics and the specific contributions of early global ethicists like Aristotle, St. Thomas Aquinas, and Immanuel

© Springer International Publishing Switzerland 2016   229
S.C. Stain et al. (eds.), *The SAGES Manual Ethics*
of Surgical Innovation, DOI 10.1007/978-3-319-27663-2_21

Kant are beyond the scope of this chapter, but in order to appreciate the need for a guideline regarding the ethical introduction of new technology, the works of John Stuart Mill and John Rawls, in particular, must be considered [2, 3]. These philosophers proposed that autonomy and self-determination are critically important concepts in health care.

Patient autonomy and self-determination are doctrines at the heart of informed consent for medical treatments and procedures. Patients have the right to make their own life choices and to receive health care free of control by others. Further, patients have the right to determine which recommended treatments and procedures they will avail themselves of without retribution by providers. In order to make these choices, patients must be informed of facts and likelihoods related to their treatment or procedure.

In the case of new technology, patient autonomy and self-determination are inexorably related to the informed consent process, as without a discussion of the new technology itself, its clinical applications, what is known and unknown, and the potential risks related not just to the procedure itself, but to the technology alone and combined with the procedure as it currently exists, consent cannot be obtained. In other words, in order for the surgeon to utilize new technologies in the treatment of patients, she/he must first understand and preserve the patient's right to self-determination by educating the patient about the new technology and allowing them to decide if they want to avail themselves of its potential benefits. At the same time, the surgeon must innovate; even in the conduct of standard procedures, there are unforeseen circumstances that mandate that the surgeon apply creativity, calling into service treatment principles ordinarily applied elsewhere. Guidance is needed, not just for the introduction of new techniques and technologies, but for their clinical applications.

The Guideline Process

The never-ending introduction and adoption of new techniques and technologies has been uncoordinated and undisciplined at times, leading to increased rates of complications in some instances [4]. SAGES leadership, through a carefully conducted Delphi process aimed at identifying priorities for minimally invasive surgery and endoscopy research, identified that two of the top ten questions to be answered were, "What is the best method for incorporating new techniques and technology for surgeons of variable levels of experience or training?" and "What are the costs associated with the introduction of new technologies and how can they be minimized?" [5]. SAGES leadership then assigned the members of the Guidelines Committee the task of researching and developing a guideline that would inform the introduction of new technologies and techniques.

The SAGES Guidelines Committee identified and reviewed pertinent literature and interviewed members of the SAGES Governing Board to gather expert consensus when published literature left knowledge gaps unaddressed (Table 21.1) [1]. Following completion of the Board surveys and interviews, the Committee set out to define terms to ensure a level of uniformity essential to this process (Table 21.2). The SAGES Guidelines Committee assesses both the quality of the evidence supporting a recommendation and the strength of the recommendation itself, according to the GRADE system (Table 21.3), using a four-tiered system for quality of evidence (**very low (+)**, **low (++)**, **moderate (+++)**, or **high (++++)**) and a two-tiered system for strengths of recommendation (**weak** or **strong**) [6].

Table 21.1. The knowledge gap in current literature, posed as questions, to be used in developing the SAGES Guideline for the introduction of new technology and techniques.

1. What is the definition of new technology and procedure?

2. What process should be followed during introduction of new technology and procedures?

3. What should be the training requirements for surgeons incorporating new devices and procedures into their practice?

4. How should surgeons be assessed for their readiness to safely implement new technology and procedures in their practice?

5. What are the criteria that should be taken into account when evaluating the value of new technology and procedures (before introduction)?

6. What outcomes should be assessed after the introduction of new technology and procedures to prove their safety and effectiveness?

7. What should be included in the consent when patients undergo new technology and procedures?

8. What should be the regulatory requirements for the introduction of new technology and procedures?

Table 21.2. Important definitions.

Technology… *synonymous with device*

Technique… *synonymous with procedure*

Modified device… *existing device, familiar to surgeon, e.g., a stapler with a new handle*

New device… *a disruptive technology, new to the surgeon*

Modified procedure… *similar to procedures the surgeon performs presently, e.g., gastric bypass to sleeve gastrectomy*

New procedure… *entirely new procedure, e.g., n POEM*

Table 21.3. Quality of evidence and strength of recommendations according to GRADE.

Quality of evidence	Definition	Symbol used
High quality	Further research is very unlikely to alter confidence in the estimate of impact	++++
Moderate quality	Further research is likely to alter confidence in the estimate of impact and may change the estimate	+++
Low quality	Further research is very likely to alter confidence in the estimate of impact and is likely to change the estimate	++
Very low quality	Any estimate of impact is uncertain	+

GRADE recommendations based on the quality of evidence for SAGES guidelines

Strong	It is very certain that benefit exceeds risk for the option considered
Weak	Risk and benefit well balanced, patients and providers faced with differing clinical situations likely would make different choices, or benefits available but not certain regarding the option considered

Adapted from Guyatt GH, Oxman AD, Vist GE, Kunz R, Falck-Ytter Y, Alonso-Coello P, et al. GRADE: an emerging consensus on rating quality of evidence and strength of recommendations. Bmj. 2008;336(7650):924–6, with permission

The Recommendations

The SAGES Guidelines Committee developed seven recommendations regarding the ethical introduction of new technologies and techniques, to serve its surgeon members, their patients, our industry partners, and administrative and other members of the health care team [1]. These are presented and discussed below.

Recommendation 1

Surgical societies should provide assessments of new technology and techniques in a timely fashion to practicing surgeons to aid their decision-making when contemplating the introduction of new technology and techniques (++, Strong).

SAGES recognizes and accepts this leadership responsibility among professional societies and, in order to promote patient autonomy and self-determination, has endeavored to create guidelines and technology assessments for use by its members as part of its moral imprimatur. With guidance from the SAGES Board, the Guidelines Committee and the Technology and Value Assessment Committee (TAVAC) provide assessment and evaluation of new technologies and techniques and publish and disseminate a variety of types of publications to achieve this end.

Recommendation 2

(A) *Surgeons considering the introduction of new technology and techniques in their practice should have device- or procedure-specific training to decrease learning curve-related complications and thus improve patient safety (+++, Strong).*

(B) *The necessary training steps depend on the degree of novelty/change and may include informal familiarization of surgeon with the device or procedure before its introduction; review of existing data/literature; the pursuit of expert input; video review of device use or procedure; practice on appropriate simulated, animate, or cadaveric training models; course participation at society meetings; proctoring or tele-proctoring of initial cases; and team training (+, Strong).*

This important recommendation conveys the ethical responsibility shared by surgeons and industry alike that obligates each to ensure that adequate training accompanies the launch of new technologies and techniques. Recognizing that some technological advances represent entirely new products while others represent minor alterations to existing products, the training process must be scalable, accounting for these differences and differences in the baseline skill-set of the surgeon. Associated training protocols must be right-sized for both the advance and for the individual surgeon pursuing facility with the new device or procedure.

Recommendation 3

While institutions, experienced centers, specialty societies, and industry all play a role in the training of surgeons in new technology and techniques, experienced centers and specialty societies have the primary responsibility for training in new procedures and devices; industry's role should be limited to new and modified devices, and all conflicts of interest should be disclosed and minimized (+, Weak).

Conflicts of interest that could influence patient care, or could appear to improperly influence patient care decisions, must be disclosed in order to maintain the public trust [7–11]. Close working relationships with industry are vital to continued growth in surgery, endoscopy, and all medical fields, but complete transparency is required so that patients, payors, and other health care constituents are able to make informed choices. Professional societies and leading medical centers must assume their roles as trainers, rather than delegating this responsibility to industry, and in these roles, must maintain an unbiased position that seeks value.

Recommendation 4

Surgeons who introduce a new device or procedure in their practice should have completed relevant surgical training, possess operating privileges in the affected organ system, and be able to address anticipated complications (++, Strong).

This recommendation is focused on a surgeon's individual responsibility to prepare for all procedures they intend to perform and for the safe and effective deployment of any new or existing technologies they plan to employ. Although health care facilities rely on credentialing processes that help assure the public that surgeons at any given facility have been vetted properly, SAGES states herein that each surgeon has a personal obligation to prepare themselves optimally for care of the patient.

Recommendation 5

For minor modifications of devices and procedures, surgeons should monitor their practice based on self-assessment. The more substantial the change in surgeons' practice and the higher the risk to the patient, the more important it is that surgeons complete a relevant didactic course and have their performance objectively assessed and their outcomes monitored by an external entity (+, Strong).

Recommendation 6

To protect their patients, surgeons should demonstrate the highest level of professionalism and exercise self-assessment and self-regulation when introducing new technology and techniques in their practice. Besides the FDA, which regulates the production and sale of new devices, institutional credentialing and/or new technology committees and the IRB should monitor their introduction in clinical practice. The introduction of novel procedures should be overseen by the credentialing committee and/or the IRB, while the role of specialty societies and new technology committees needs further assessment (+, Strong).

Recommendations 5 and 6 build on the theme that patient protection is best assured through transparent and ongoing assessment. Surgeons are innovators, researchers, scientists, and as such maintain an approach to patient care that seeks optimal outcomes. Adopting minor procedural changes might require little more than informal training and periodic review of aggregated procedures, whereas the incorporation of major changes or entirely new procedures will require formal study, and when appropriate, Institutional Review Board or other oversight. Regardless of institutional mandates, surgeons should objectively assess their results and patient outcomes whenever new or modified procedures are employed.

Recommendation 7

The effectiveness compared to alternatives, the cost, patient outcomes, and the safety profile of new technology and techniques should always be assessed prior to and after their introduction. Other parameters such as existing and required resources; benefits to patients, surgeons, and hospitals; existing or anticipated volume of use; barriers to adoption; and whether the anticipated benefits prove real after introduction should also be considered, especially for significant changes in devices and procedures, besides minor modifications (+++, Strong).

It is the ethical responsibility for health care providers to consider the comparative effectiveness of available treatments and to assess the value represented by new procedures and technologies as well as modifications to existing techniques and technologies. In considering the adoption of modified or new techniques and technologies, the surgeon must consider available resources and determine if they are sufficient to support the launch of something new, and its sustained use for all subsequent patients should its results be promising.

Conclusions

The Society of American Gastrointestinal and Endoscopic Surgeons (SAGES), regarded as the premier membership organization for general surgeons worldwide, approaches the guidance of its members, their patients, and other health care constituents through education, a central precept of its mission. Guidelines provide a framework of recommendations for clinical practice, training, and in the case of new technologies and techniques, their ethical introduction.

In considering the diversity of patients, surgeons, and environments where new technologies and techniques will be utilized, SAGES has taken up the task to create a guideline that provides ethical direction, a challenge that few other professional societies have embraced. As SAGES, the organization, has recognized and accepted its responsibility to guide the world of surgery with technology and value assessments, and guidelines, it too has charged its members with creating and maintaining a patient-first approach wherever new technologies are deployed, with patient safety as priority one. Unlike some organizational approaches that seek to paint all new developments with the same brush, SAGES, through this guideline document, recognizes that the approach must be scalable, the magnitude of required education and experience directly related to the magnitude of change associated with the new technology or technique. This approach ensures that patient safety is prioritized, yet does not unreasonably restrict patient access to new treatment modalities.

This SAGES guideline also calls on experienced medical centers, their staff surgeons, and professional societies in the aggregate to respond to the challenge of educating surgeons in new technologies and techniques. In the past, much of this educational need was fulfilled by industry, and while guidance from industry representatives often is quite useful, especially in the case of new or modified devices during their initial use, this guideline espouses an approach that puts industry in a more peripheral role and surgical educators in the primary role of disseminating advances in surgical care, to limit potential conflicts of interest [7, 8, 11, 12].

No matter where a surgeon learns to use a new device, or to perform a new procedure, transparency in discussions with patients, self-motivation to receive appropriate training and education, enlisting the oversight of the Institutional Review Board when appropriate, and engaging in continual self-assessment regarding performance with the new technique all are hallmarks of a responsible deployment of new technologies and techniques. Along with safety monitoring, cost and effectiveness monitoring remains an important component of this process, and the SAGES guideline recommends that cost and utility should be assessed prior to introduction, and after adoption, extracting value where possible.

In considering the message of any guideline, whether produced by SAGES or by one of the several other professional societies that publish useful evidence-based guidelines, it is as important to consider what the guideline does not say as it is to consider the recommendations that are made. The SAGES guideline does not say that surgeons cannot partner with industry to advance patient care; transparency is critical, as is a patient-centric approach to all relationships, but collaboration with industry has resulted in many advances that benefit patients on a daily basis, and these relationships continue to be important venues for the development of surgical advancements. The guideline does not convey the message that novel techniques and new technologies cannot or should not be developed and introduced. While we are cautioned that value is important, as is ongoing assessment, there is great opportunity to improve patient outcomes and enhance health care value through new developments.

Finally, the guideline does not advocate that the processes used to deploy new technologies and techniques be onerous or stifling. Rather, SAGES and its Guidelines Committee have advocated that a rational, scalable approach be used, where the magnitude of process is directly related to the magnitude of change encountered with the new device or procedure compared to the existing technologies and approaches. Using a scalable deployment model is very patient-first and allows the greatest number of patients access to new technologies and techniques, through safe deployments that contribute to outcomes databases, and search for value in future episodes of care.

References

1. Stefanidis D, Fanelli RD, Price R, Richardson W, Committee SG. SAGES guidelines for the introduction of new technology and techniques. Surg Endosc. 2014;28(8):2257–71.
2. Schweigert FJ. The priority of justice: a framework approach to ethics in program evaluation. Eval Program Plann. 2007;30(4):394–9.
3. Gillon R. Autonomy and the principle of respect for autonomy. Br Med J. 1985;290(6484):1806–8.
4. Barone JE, Lincer RM. Correction: a prospective analysis of 1518 laparoscopic cholecystectomies. N Engl J Med. 1991;325(21):1517–8.
5. Stefanidis D, Montero P, Urbach DR, Qureshi A, Perry K, Bachman SL, et al. SAGES research agenda in gastrointestinal and endoscopic surgery: updated results of a Delphi study. Surg Endosc. 2014;28(10):2763–71.
6. Guyatt GH, Oxman AD, Vist GE, Kunz R, Falck-Ytter Y, Alonso-Coello P, et al. GRADE: an emerging consensus on rating quality of evidence and strength of recommendations. BMJ. 2008;336(7650):924–6.
7. Morrow DR. When technologies makes good people do bad things: another argument against the value-neutrality of technologies. Sci Eng Ethics. 2014;20(2):329–43.
8. Van Haute A. Managing perceived conflicts of interest while ensuring the continued innovation of medical technology. J Vasc Surg. 2011;54(3 Suppl):31S–3.
9. Frequently asked questions regarding the revised Advanced Medical Technology Association (AdvaMed) Code of Ethics on Interactions with Health Care Professionals. Optometry. 2009;80(5):262–6.
10. Orfanos CE. From Hippocrates to modern medicine. J Eur Acad Dermatol Venereo. 2007;21(6):852–8.
11. Sachdeva AK. Acquiring skills in new procedures and technology: the challenge and the opportunity. Arch Surg. 2005;140(4):387–9.
12. Holsinger Jr JW, Beaton B. Physician professionalism for a new century. Clin Anat. 2006;19(5):473–9.

22. Training Physicians in Innovation

Dan Azagury, James Wall, Anji Wall, and Thomas Krummel

Barriers to Medical Innovation

The great surgeon innovators of a distant (or not so distant) past are greatly revered in our medical textbooks: Doctors Theodore Kocher, Thomas Fogarty, or Norman Shumway are seen as pioneers, and their innovations, whether surgical or technical, have revolutionized entire medical fields. So why is innovation not a cornerstone of current medical education?

As most things medical, this is likely multifactorial. There is a clear lack of innovation curriculum in medical school, both in the United States and abroad. With the increase in medical knowledge and medical subspecialization, medical schools curricula face no lack in education material and topics needing to be covered. So why is innovation often not a priority in these programs? Medical schools aim to prepare students to become successful doctors: Either clinically, in research or both. Innovation is neither part of our clinical practice, nor an academically recognized research field. So should innovation be a third option? Should it remain a hobby for a few heretics? We would argue it should simply be part of both: Innovation should be part of our clinical practice: MDs have a unique insight into all the shortcomings of our medical practice and that unique knowledge should not be discarded. It should be put to use in order to identify unmet clinical needs and drive innovation from the bedside. And in order to be adequately encouraged, innovation should also be adequately regarded: it should also be part of academia, on par with any other research field.

S.C. Stain et al. (eds.), *The SAGES Manual Ethics of Surgical Innovation*, DOI 10.1007/978-3-319-27663-2_22

Furthermore, innovation could be easily applied to any academic medical specialty. These could easily integrate the new physician-innovators among physician-scientists and scientist-physicians [3]. One of the barriers to integration of innovation in academia is the "inherent conflict of interest with industry." There is widespread belief in academia that developing novel medical devices is an inherently commercial project. It is often viewed as an entryway for industry into universities by way of financially supporting projects and influencing research. However, while the relationship between clinicians and industry has the potential for conflict of interest when a device is at the commercial stage, the development phase is very different. There is no more reason for confliction at the early stages of device development than for other biomedical research fields.

The Innovation Mindset

In order for physicians to incorporate innovation in their practice, they should be trained in innovation (acquire the skillset). As we will explain in this chapter, innovation can be taught, just like cell culture or RNA assays. But physicians also need to have an "innovating mindset." In our view, that does not need to be taught in medical school. It only needs not to be crushed by medical education. Indeed, the basis of current medical education is evidence. Evidence-based medicine requires current best practices to be based upon longstanding and extensive pre-existing research. This is obviously commendable and a very positive teaching system to ensure high-quality training. However, this method will, by definition, discard any treatment, approach, or management that has not been demonstrated by clinical trials. By doing this, the message conveyed to our students is that current treatments are to be regarded as "ideal" as they have scientifically demonstrated their worth. It does not encourage students to question the treatments and method in a critical way. However, young individuals will often have a very critical and curious mind, questioning each new piece of information they encounter. Future doctors would likely be more innovative, if their curiosity and questioning was not rejected but encouraged. If we encourage our students to ask "why" and we challenge them to find better solutions than the existing ones, they will keep their curiosity alive through medical school and into their careers.

Acquiring the Skillset

Since the times of Dr. Kocher, medical technologies have grown significantly more complex. This complexity is not only technological, but also environmental. Developing and commercializing medical devices requires overcoming multiple hurdles: what regulatory pathway is required in the USA for the device to be FDA cleared or approved, or CE marked in Europe? How to secure intellectual property? What will be required to demonstrate efficacy? What are the possible engineering challenges and how can they be averted? How will the device be commercialized?

The aspects mentioned above are completely foreign to most physicians and definitely not taught in medical school. And these aspects cannot be discarded "for later"; they need to be taken into account early on in the process of innovation. If only because funding such an endeavor is already difficult enough that investors will not finance promising devices if they see multiple major barriers in the development road ahead. Programs exist however to fill that gap and teach innovation. These programs are flourishing across universities around the world: The Stanford Biodesign Program was created for that purpose nearly 15 years ago to teach physicians and engineers the process of medtech innovation [4, 5] (Fig. 22.1).

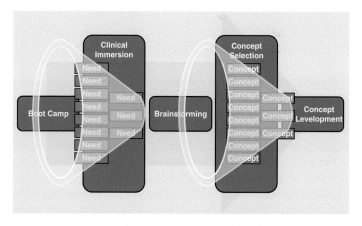

Fig. 22.1. Core Biodesign Process which consists of boot camp, needs identification, needs filtration, concept generation, concept filtration, and implementation of leading concept(s). (© Stanford University Biodesign Program, used with permission.).

It is currently available in multiple formats, including a "flagship" 10-month full-time fellowship. This is a team-based, process-driven experience. It combines theoretical lectures and teaching, with a real-life experience of being driven through the entire process of innovation. Teams of four fellows with diverse backgrounds in medicine, engineering, and business will be created specifically for the duration of the fellowship. They will first be subject to a month-long boot camp, heavy in lectures and expert presentations. Courses include intellectual property, regulatory pathway, market overview, funding sources, and mechanisms, etc. Then, teams are paired up with a medical department in the adjacent hospital in order to directly observe patient care and identify unmet clinical needs. The teams will then follow the entire process consisting of needs identification, needs filtration, concept generation, concept filtration, and early stage implementation of the inventions. They will often keep pursuing their innovation after the fellowship is over.

This setup allows fellows not only to understand medtech innovation, but also to live it firsthand. It also provides a unique process and a unique environment for the fellows to identify problems across a wide array of clinical settings and be completely free to invent any solution they deem is most likely to solve the need they identified. We think this provides fellows the required skillset and network but also encourages them to completely adopt their creative mindset and face no limitations to their imagination.

Conflicts of Interest in Medtech Innovation

The primary ethical issues that arise with physician entrepreneurs are those surrounding questions of conflicts of interest. A commonly used definition of conflict of interest is "a set of conditions in which professional judgment concerning a primary interest tends to be unduly influenced by a secondary interest" [6–8]. This definition identifies the primary interest as professional, allows for the secondary interest to be of any nature, and incorporates the notion of undue influence, indicating that interests only conflict when the secondary interest unduly influences professional judgment about the primary interest. There are a few clarifications that improve this definition of conflict of interest. First, the undue influence created by the secondary interest does not have to be real; it can be perceived. Second, the secondary interest is not necessarily illegitimate; it is just not the interest that has priority. Finally, a conflict of interest does not require intention (i.e., the individual with the conflict does not have to be aware of the bias created by the secondary interest). A more precise definition states that a conflict of interest occurs when a primary professional interest either appears to be or is unduly influenced, consciously or unconsciously, by a secondary interest.

Conflicts of interest are problematic because they undermine the perception of the public toward the institution or individual with the real or perceived conflict [9]. If the public perception of the physician entrepreneur is undermined by real or perceived bias created by the physician's secondary interests, trust in the individual will be damaged, affecting their ability to care for patients. Furthermore, conflicts of interest can degrade trust in entire institutions, so they can have effects outside of the individual physician's practice.

Defining Interests

The first step to determining whether or not a conflict of interest exists is to identify the primary professional interest. The primary interest of physician entrepreneurs in their clinical role is to fulfill their fiduciary duty to patients. Next, the competing secondary interest must be identified. There are many secondary interests that physician entrepreneurs have to manage. These include financial gain from clinical use of their devices, professional gain through publication about their outcomes, and deeply invested personal interest in seeing the products they have designed be successful in the clinical setting. Each of these can create a real or perceived influence on the primary interest of patient care.

Managing Conflicts of Interest

There are three primary ways in which conflicts of interest are managed: avoidance, disclosure, and education. Avoidance is the most straightforward way of dealing with conflicts of interest. It involves recognizing that something has the potential to create a conflict of interest and eliminating it [9]. It is the most effective way of dealing with conflicts of interest because it completely eliminates the potential for either real or perceived bias to be created by the secondary interest. However, avoidance is only possible when the secondary interest is unnecessary, and can be eliminated without creating significant negative consequences. In the field of device design, even if financial and professional interests were eliminated completely, it would be impossible to eliminate the physician entrepreneur's personal interest in the device. The main exception to this statement is if the device would be used by other physicians, in which case the physician entrepreneur would not have to be involved in clinical trials or in using the device for patient care.

Disclosure is a second method for handling conflicts of interest. The purpose of disclosure is to allow the patient to discount the provided information by some amount, based on the type and extent of the conflict. It allows the patient to make an informed decision and to opt out or change expectations [10–12]. Disclosure can be problematic because it assumes that the conflict is recognizable, and that the person to whom the information is disclosed can use it to determine if there is bias and to what extent the information is being biased [8, 11, 13]. With disclosure, the responsibility is placed on the patient to judge the validity of the information [9]. Moreover, disclosure does nothing to control or resolve the conflict, but merely "sanitizes" it [11–13]. While not perfect, disclosure is an appropriate part of conflict of interest management when secondary interests are both recognizable and necessary, which is the case with physician entrepreneurs. It is essential that physician entrepreneurs develop their disclosure process with their employers and legal council so as to ensure that they are providing adequate information for patients to be able to effectively use it to determine bias and make decisions based on the disclosure.

Education is a third approach to managing conflicts of interest. Education means teaching individuals about secondary interests that can cause bias and presenting strategies to minimize the effects of these interests on their behavior. Physician entrepreneurs must be conscious of the myriad secondary interests that can bias their management of patients and to make efforts to minimize these interests when possible. This involves ensuring that compensation for device design or consultation is not exorbitant and that professional advancement is not solely reliant on device success among other things.

Aligning Interests

Much of the literature on conflicts of interest makes the assumption that secondary interests are either illegitimate or diametrically opposed to a primary interest. Physician entrepreneurs have the opportunity to work against this assumption. While the primary clinical interest of physician entrepreneurs is to care for their patients, their primary interest as innovators is to create devices that improve the care of patients in general. Therefore, their interest in the individual patient is most often aligned with their interest in helping patients on a larger scale. The art of being a physician entrepreneur is determining what secondary interests exist, eliminating these interests when possible, disclosing them in a way that allows patients to make informed decisions regarding their care, and educating oneself on how to minimize real and perceived bias from these interests. Knowledge of legal and institutional standards regarding conflicts of interest is essential for success in this realm.

Teamology

There is no absolute formula for a design team. Two things are clear from 15 years of experience in the Biodesign process. First, a team of individually accomplished individuals who cannot collaborate typically leads to disaster. On the contrary, a team of individual who can come together to exploit individual strengths and minimize conflict is able to develop projects with real impact on patients. Research from the Hasso Plattner institute confirms this observation by showing that the common wisdom of combining individuals with diverse cognitive abilities alone does not correlate with team performance. It is in fact "social sensitivity," the cognitive ability to relate to other team members' problem solving preferences that correlate to improved performance [14].

Team building plays a significant role in the Biodesign program as it has evolved. The first part of team building is an a priori attempt to fill the team with individuals that have diverse backgrounds and compatible personalities. We believe the backgrounds necessary for medical innovation teams include a physician member with clinical experience, an engineer member with research experience, and an industry member with business, and regulatory or other medical technology experience. In addition to background, the personalities of each team member should be considered. Again, there is no formula, but we seek complementary personalities of the organizer, the thinker, the builder, and the clinician.

Physician Roles in Biodesign

Medical technology translation generally follows two distinct pathways. The first pathway involves "Technology Push" where scientists develop deep expertise in a specific area and then follow investigation protocols that expand knowledge. Such programs can lead to discoveries of transformative technology that must then be applied to an appropriate problem. The clinical application is occasionally immediately obvious with immense implications; however, more often than not the application of a laboratory-discovered technology to patient care is not obvious. The investigators must then begin the arduous process of fitting a technology to a clinical problem.

An alternative approach to the development of medical technology is "Technology Pull." This approach is based on design thinking as embodied by the work of Tom and David Kelley at IDEO [15]. The process begins with observing and defining the need of the customer. In healthcare, the customer point of view typically begins with the patient. The Biodesign process as pioneered at Stanford takes design thinking principles and adds analysis of the intricacies of the healthcare system in the initial evaluation of the need including value, regulatory requirements, intellectual property, and workflow. By fully understanding the problem, the market, the stakeholder incentives, and the development pathway of what a good solution requires, one can make informed decisions on which projects warrant time and effort with the most chance of success.

The Biodesign process has proven successful at Stanford using "Technology Pull" as measured by the development of over thirty start-up companies, multiple approved medical devices on the market, and ultimately over 350,000 patients treated as of 2015. Perhaps the greatest validation of the program has been the rapid growth of similar programs in the United States and beyond. At the core of this success is constant involvement of clinicians on the design teams, strong relationships with clinical departments to expose teams to the breadth of clinical problems worth solving, and clinical mentorship for teams through concept development. With growth of design thinking for medical technology, the question arises of how many physicians should be trained in this methodology?

We believe that exposure to design thinking is valuable to all physicians who seek a better way to treat patients. Even for physicians working on fundamental scientific discoveries, the ability to apply the Biodesign process post hoc to a technology they discover can shorten the timeframe to success patient implementation. The full year-long fellowship is only suitable for those who plan to make innovation a significant part of their career. For physicians who seek initial exposure to the Biodesign process, faculty fellowships and executive courses are now being offered that limit time commitment while maintain exposure to the full cycle of Biodesign innovation.

References

1. Krummel TM, Gertner M, Makower J, Milroy C, Gurtner G, Woo R, et al. Inventing our future: training the next generation of surgeon innovators. Semin Pediatr Surg. 2006;15:309–18.
2. Health technology assessment (Winchester, England).
3. Majmudar MD, Harrington MRA, Graham FNJBG, McConnell FMV. The clinician innovator: a novel career path in academic medicine. In Press.
4. Yock PG, Brinton TJ, Zenios SA. Teaching biomedical technology innovation as a discipline. Sci Transl Med. 2011. 3:92cm18.
5. Brinton TJ, Kurihara CQ, Camarillo DB, Pietzsch JB, Gorodsky J, Zenios SA, et al. Outcomes from a postgraduate biomedical technology innovation training program: the first 12 years of Stanford biodesign. Ann Biomed Eng. 2013;41:1803–10.
6. Holmes DR, Firth BG, James A, Winslow R, Hodgson PK, Gamble GL, et al. Conflict of interest. Am Heart J. 2004;147:228–37.
7. Stossel TP. Regulating academic-industrial research relationships – solving problems or stifling progress? N Engl J Med. 2005;353:1060–5.
8. Thompson DF. Understanding financial conflicts of interest. N Engl J Med. 1993; 329:573–6.
9. Parascandola M. A turning point for conflicts of interest: the controversy over the National Academy of Sciences' first conflicts of interest disclosure policy. J Clin Oncol. 2007;25:3774–9.
10. Tonelli MR. Conflict of interest in clinical practice. Chest. 2007;132:664–70.
11. Foster RS. Conflicts of interest: recognition, disclosure, and management. J Am Coll Surg. 2003;196:505–17.
12. Moore DA, Cain DM, Loewenstein G, Bazerman MH. Conflicts of interest: challenges and solutions in business, law, medicine, and public policy. New York: Cambridge University Press; 2005.
13. Brennan TA, Rothman DJ, Blank L, Blumenthal D, Chimonas SC, Cohen JJ, et al. Health industry practices that create conflicts of interest: a policy proposal for academic medical centers. JAMA. 2006;295:429–33.
14. Plattner H, Meinel C, Leifer L. Design thinking research. Springer Science & Business Media; 2012. New York, NY. pp. 189–209.
15. Kelley D, Kelley T. Unleashing the creative potential within us all. HarperCollins: Creative Confidence; 2013. p. 21–8.

23. Fundamentals of Medical Ethics

Arthur L. Rawlings

It is practically impossible to go through medical training, or even just to be around the medical field, without a discussion or two along the way about the proper course of action in a difficult medical situation. The challenging medical ethical questions are legion. The pressure of time may drive one past the initial questions of how to arrive at an answer to an ethical dilemma on to the concluding question, "What should we do?" This chapter is about those initial questions and asks what are some of the principles involved and what is a process that can be used to arrive at the answer to a difficult medical ethical challenge. In short, it is on the fundamentals of medical ethics.

Fundamentals refer to the principles by which decisions are made, not the decisions themselves. The field of applied ethics is concerned about the decisions. Pick up any major applied ethics textbook and there will be chapters on such topics as euthanasia, in vitro fertilization, cloning, and allocation of scarce resources. A closer reading of the text will reveal the approach by which the authors arrive at their conclusions. It is those approaches that are of concern in this chapter.

It is equally important to recognize that this is a chapter on medical ethics. There are other ethical domains worthy of discussion such as business ethics, engineering ethics, and legal ethics. Each has its own unique set of questions as well as nuanced approaches to answer those questions raised. Though some of the discussion here is applicable to ethics in general, the focus will be on its application to medicine in particular.

One final clarification is needed. This chapter is about medical practice and less about medical research. The broad-brush stroke is that medical practice is the application of generalized medical knowledge to a specific clinical situation, whereas medical research is using clinical situations to generate generalizable knowledge. It is the direction of information flow that delineates the two. Medical research raises its own unique set of questions. What constitutes a proper informed consent for

© Springer International Publishing Switzerland 2016
S.C. Stain et al. (eds.), *The SAGES Manual Ethics
of Surgical Innovation*, DOI 10.1007/978-3-319-27663-2_23

research? What should the relationship be between the group studied and the benefits they receive from the study? How is research conducted with vulnerable populations such as children? When is the risk of research not worth the reward? Other chapters in this text will have a greater focus on the ethics of medical research.

Three Basic Domains

There are three basic domains of inquiry into ethics—descriptive, normative, and metaethical [1]. Descriptive ethics is the discipline of explaining and describing moral phenomena. Historians, anthropologists, and sociologists typically do this type of investigation. Their work describes ethical behaviors and beliefs of individuals or groups of people. It is a statement of what is. How are organs allocated for transplant in the United States? What does the majority believe about voluntary passive euthanasia? How does the process of informed consent for surgery occur in most hospitals? How does that process differ if the consent is for research?

Normative ethics investigates what should be done. It is prescriptive, not descriptive. This is what people are usually after when they ask, "What should I do?" The question is not so much what is everyone doing, but what should everyone be doing. Normative ethics would not ask how organs are allocated for transplant in the United States. It would ask how should they be allocated. Normative ethics is the main focus of the discussion that follows.

Metaethics asks the most basic questions of morality itself. What does it mean to be good? What is justice? How is a person autonomous? Is it right for people to refuse to donate their organs after they have died? What is the relationship between the person who was recently alive and the deceased body? These are more foundational questions that will rarely be touched on here.

Four Major Theories

There are four major theories that one should be aware of when discussing medical ethics. There are more that can be discussed, but these have made a significant contribution to ethics in general and medical ethics in particular. Each theory has its strengths and weakness. None is the panacea for medical ethical dilemmas, but each one can be a part of the solution to such dilemmas.

Utilitarianism

Choosing to act in such a way to maximize happiness is an approach to medical ethical decision-making known as utilitarianism. Its two greatest historical proponents are Jeremy Bentham (1748–1832) and John Stuart Mill (1806–1873) [2]. This ethical system has two basic forms. In act-utilitarianism, a person should act so as to produce the greatest good over evil with consideration for everyone involved. This approach focuses on the consequences of a given act. What its utility is for generating good. More accurately it is to consider several different acts for a given situation, tally the consequences of each, and chooses the act that is most favorable for creating good. In rule-utilitarianism, a person should act upon the rules that would produce the greatest good. Rather than just looking at each individual act, rule-utilitarianism asks if there are specific rules that one should follow that would generally create the greatest good. For example, the rule to maintain physician-patient confidentiality could be employed by a rule-utilitarian as this generally brings about more happiness in society that breaking that confidentiality without reason. In both utilitarianism approaches, the utility of an act to bring about the desired good is the most important component of the theory.

This theory has several commendable features. It recognizes that actions are not performed in a vacuum but usually have community consequences. The surgeon in a massive casualty situation that empties the blood bank on one person may have helped one patient but took limited valuable resources away from many that could have potentially been helped had the resources been allocated differently. Saving one life may not have brought about as much good as saving ten lives. Secondly, utilitarianism does recognize that the end matters. Medical futility rests upon this concept. An exploratory laparotomy may be done in one setting and not in another just because of the medically expected outcome. The action of the laparotomy would essentially be the same in either case, but the expected outcome informs the decision of whether or not to take the patient to surgery.

As good as utilitarianism is, certain issues are raised. The primary issue is how to make the calculus to compare one good with another. How is good quantified? Would saving one patient for ten years be worth taking one year away from nine other patients giving a net gain of one patient year? Calculations like this are difficult. When the National Highway Traffic Safety Administration calculated that a human life was worth $200,725 in their 1972 report, the Ford Motor Company used that figure to calculate the cost-benefit analysis of upgrading their Pinto's gas tank.

The cost of the upgrade was 2.77 times higher than the cost of not upgrading so the company decided to leave 12.5 million vehicles on the road without any changes [3]. For some reason, though, the public thought that there was something fundamentally wrong with that calculation. The second and more basic question is what is the good that is to be maximized? Is it pure pleasure? Are other goods such as friendship, loyalty, and community more important than happiness? Is it overall life expectancy with little regard to the quality of life? This struggle is played out in intensive care units on a daily basis in the United States as families wrestle with continuing aggressive therapy or moving to comfort measures. Finally, how does one determine all the foreseen consequences? How significant does the immediate consequence have to be to be included in the calculation? How far in the future does one have to look? Is it ok to exhaust all limited resources in one generation with little regard to the next generation or should the happiness of those not yet born be considered? There are no crystal balls handed out in medical school. Many consequences are unknown or unforeseen, and they may be the most important ones for the calculation had they been known.

Kantian Theories

While utilitarianism in its various forms focuses on the consequences of an action, deontological (Greek: deon—"duty" and logia—"discourse") approaches focus on the duty of the act itself. Immanuel Kant (1724–1804) was a major proponent of this concept with his categorical imperative [4]. He stressed that people should not be viewed as a means, but as an end. This categorical imperative is more likely known by the concept that one should act in such a way that one could will that the act be universal. Or, as it has been simply put, "Do unto others as you were the others." There are several variations of this concept of duty, but they will all be lumped under Kant's name here.

This ethical theory has several commendable qualities. First, it resonates with ordinary moral thinking. Do not lie. Do not steal. Do not kill. These acts in themselves are generally thought of as universal and have been taught to most of us since childhood. Secondly, this system is very duty bound. You are under obligation to perform the act just as anyone else would be if in that situation. The corollary is that people have rights. There is the duty not to lie because people have the right to the truth. One should not kill because people have the right to life. Finally, this approach is very normative. What should be done is what anyone in that situation should do.

Kantian approaches fall short in a couple areas. The first of which is that it focuses on the action devoid of emotion. There seems to be something missing when a surgeon performs surgery on a patient because it is needed, but does not want to perform it to help the patient. Secondly, it does not help adjudicate between competing duties. The surgeon who is not on call but is requested in the very late afternoon to do a laparoscopic appendectomy in a good friend with acute appendicitis has wrestled with this issue of competing duties when she has also promised her daughter that she would leave on time to attend her daughter's basketball game. Should she fulfill her duty to her daughter or to her friend?

Virtue Ethics

In utilitarianism and Kantian approaches, the emphasis, respectively, is upon the act's outcome or the act itself. In virtue ethics, the focus is on the agent of the action. The principle is that the virtuous person will do what is right when faced with a moral choice. If this is so, then the focus should be upon what types of virtues one should have and what vices one should avoid to be a virtuous person. This ancient approach, coming from Plato and Aristotle, praised such traits as honesty, integrity, compassion, and courage. These virtues can be acquired through training in the same manner a person acquires the skill to play an instrument—practice, practice, practice. Acting out the virtues is not enough. One must also have the morally appropriate desire to act as well. This is an added dimension to utilitarianism and Kantian approaches. In these two systems, a person can have the capacity to do the right thing, intend to do it, and actually do it while all the time wishing to be able to avoid doing it. Utilitarianism and Kantian approaches allows one to ask, "Do you want a surgeon who is good in the operating room or one who has good bedside manners?" Virtue ethics sees this as a false dichotomy. It demands that something is missing if a person does not have an appropriate desire wed to the appropriate act.

As good as virtue ethics is at addressing the concern that the agent is as valuable as the act in a moral activity, it still falls short of a complete theory. The first concern is what constitutes a virtue. What is so good about honesty? Could lying be a virtue? To say that honesty is a virtue and lying a vice because that is what virtuous people do becomes circular reasoning. Asking questions like these moves beyond virtue ethics to metaethics, the very foundational questions of morality. Virtue ethics may avoid metaethics and call upon Kantian approaches to uncover the duties one is to perform. Either approach demonstrates that virtue ethics is not the panacea for medical ethics. No universally accepted list of virtues and vices has been collected by which all practice medicine. Yet, virtue ethics does add a component to the other approaches already discussed. It demands that the desire be matched up with the deed.

Secondly, even if a universally accepted list of virtues and vices is produced, the theory provides little guidance about how to act when two virtues are in conflict. The Tarasoff decision is a classic example. A patient told a psychologist that he is going to kill an individual as soon as the opportunity arises. What is the psychologist to do? Is he to uphold the virtue of confidentiality and trust to his client and not warn the threatened individual? Or is he to exercise compassion and tell the individual of the threat? Virtue ethics would say that the virtuous person would do the right thing in that situation, but it is easy to conceive that the course of action would differ depending on which virtuous person was placed in that situation. Even the legal opinion is split along these two lines, indicating that this is a very difficult legal and moral dilemma to work through [5, 6].

Principalism

It should be clear that these three classic approaches—utilitarianism, Kantian approaches, and virtue ethics—have contributed to medical ethics, but none of them has become the accepted dominant theory. A newer approach has gained a significant foothold in the field of medical ethics. Principalism, formalized in the Belmont Report [7] and espoused by one of the most widely used textbooks in biomedical ethics [8], asserts that there is no foundational ethical theory universally accepted upon which to base decisions, but there is a generally accepted group of principles that can be put into service for deciding a course of action in medical ethics. The three dominant principles are autonomy, beneficence, and justice.

Autonomy

Autonomy, the right of self-governance, is one of the primary principles accepted in medical ethics today. It is born from the philosophical perspective that individuals have intrinsic value and is bolstered from Kant's idea that people are ends in themselves. This principle is respected every time a surgeon engages a patient in the process of informed consent for surgery. This seems simple, but there are various views on autonomy and constraints that should be in place. One view is that autonomy is just self-determination. This libertarian approach is the most open view with the least constraints placed upon the individual. At its most basic, a person can do what he or she wants. A second view is that autonomy is self-determination coupled with rationality. This liberal view constrains the first view with reasoned determination. A person can do what he or she wants as long as it is rational. This raises the whole question of rationality, but that is beyond the discussion here. Suffice it to say, this view requires reason behind the self-determination. Finally, the communitarian approach is that self-determination must have moral content. This approach recognizes that decisions for self-determination are not made in a vacuum. Actions of self-determination must take into account the effects on others and can be constrained by those effects [9].

As with all these principles, autonomy is only part of the conversation. The classical example is the dilemma of respecting a Jehovah's Witness expressed will to refuse a blood transfusion when one would be reasonably necessary to sustain life. It seems reasonable for one with that conviction to make that self-determination, but what if that person is making that decision for a 3-year-old son?

Beneficence and Nonmaleficence

The second principle, beneficence, is seeking the welfare of the patient. A major goal of medicine is to alleviate human suffering and to instill hope that a patient's life goals can be actualized, or at least attained to the highest level medically possible. The negative of beneficence, nonmaleficence, is expressed in the maxim *primum non nocere*, above all do no harm. This principle has had a long and rich history in the medical community, though the exact origins are debated. Beneficence and nonmaleficence are sometimes discussed separately. They will be kept together here for the sake of simplicity.

This principle has been broken down into four possible concepts [10]. First, a physician should not inflict harm or do evil to a patient. This is captured in the ancient dictum of *primum non nocere* and is solidly entrenched in medical ethics. Secondly, a physician should prevent future harm to a patient. A surgeon recommending a laparoscopic cholecystectomy to a reasonably good surgical candidate after a couple bouts of right upper quadrant pain from cholelithiasis but who is in no pain now in the clinic is exercising this concept of beneficence. The act of surgery prevents the patient future pain and suffering. Thirdly, a physician should alleviate pain and suffering. This was the primary if not sole perspective of medicine for centuries until the historically recent emphasis on preventative care. The patient saw a doctor because he was sick and wanted to get better. A patient had a disease (Old French: desaise—lack of ease) and wanted a state of ease (comfort, leisure). Finally, the physician should promote good. The required duty of this last element is more debated. The bariatric surgeon who, out of her accepted obligation to number three above, does a laparoscopic appendectomy for acute appendicitis in a patient with a BMI of 43 who cannot pay may not be duty bound to perform a Roux-en-Y gastric bypass in that same patent even if the patient requests it later.

Justice

The final principle discussed here is justice. This is the recognition that medicine is usually not practiced in isolation but in a society. Justice asks what is fair for individuals of a society; what does the individual owe the society, and what does society owe the individual? When dialysis machines were exceedingly expensive and not readily available for all who would benefit, the decision of who gets access to the equipment is one of justice. Organ allocation is the same. How should these scarce resources be distributed and to whom?

Justice is a simple concept—equals should be treated as equals and unequals as unequals. There is general agreement with the statement. That is why justice is one of the fundamental principles. However, it does not tell how to determine who are equals and who are not. Usually, the focus is not on being equal in all aspects. There is usually some relevant aspect that is being considered in determining equality. The controversy is over what are the relevant aspects in a given situation.

Once the determination of who is equal has been done, the question of justice is how resources should be shared or withheld from equal individuals. Should each person have an equal share? Should goods be distributed according to individual need? Should free market forces play a role in goods distribution? Does a person's contribution to society have any bearing on how goods are distributed? Anyone who has participated in the lifeboat exercise of trying to determine who stays in the boat and who does not when resources will not sustain everyone has wrestled with this issue of justice. Anyone who has questioned whether or not enormous medical resources should be expended on heroic, life-saving procedures to benefit a few when those resources could have been used in more mundane manners to benefit many has entertained this principle of justice.

The goal of this chapter is to outline some of the fundamentals of medical ethics. Four normative approaches have been discussed. The heart of utilitarianism is the utility of an act. The course chosen should bring about the greatest good. Kantian approaches hold that the act itself is the determining factor. One has a duty to do that which any person in that context should do. Virtue ethics focuses on the agent of the action. A good and just person will do the right thing with the right motive. Principalism moves away from grounding medical ethics in one universal concept. Instead, it searches for widely accepted principles that can form the framework for a conversation about medical ethics. Three of the most commonly accepted principles are autonomy, beneficence, and justice. All of these theories contribute to our moral conversation. None has become the widely accepted theory to the exclusion of the others.

A Process Toward a Decision

Where do we go from here? While none of the four theories has become dominant in the field of medical ethics, each one can provide concepts for medical ethical discussions. When faced with a medical ethical dilemma, a series of steps can be employed to make a decision of how to move forward.

The first step is to uncover how all these theories apply to the dilemma. Consider the surgeon offering to use new technology in a patient for the first time. The FDA has recently approved this technology for this condition, but the surgeon has never used it before. She is familiar and skilled with the traditional approach, but wants to offer this new technology to her patients. What are some of the ethical issues involved?

Utilitarianism asks if the old or new approach brings about the greatest good, though there are several goods to consider. Which approach is more likely to help patients with this disease? Does the introduction of this new technology place such a significant resource burden on the health care system that the good of this one patient population is overshadowed by the shared burden to the system? Does the use of the new technology bring little added benefit to the patient, but brings significant academic or marketing advantage to the surgeon?

Kantian approaches want to know what duties the surgeon has to the patient. She is to alleviate pain and suffering, which can be accomplished by either course of action. She is also to be truthful, but what all does the patient have to be told? Does the patient need to know that she has never used this technology in a human before? Must the patient know about all approaches if this approach has already received FDA approval for this disease?

Virtue ethics asks why the surgeon is entertaining the use of the new technology. Does she have a strong desire to help the patient and believe that the new approach could potentially bring about a better outcome? Has she purchased stock in the company and wants to use this technology to support her financial portfolio as much as possible? Is she interested in adopting the new technology because she is losing business to her competitor who is employing it in an aggressive marketing scheme even though it brings little or no benefit to the patient?

Principalism adds to this conversation by focusing on the patient's autonomy, beneficence, and justice. Is the patient informed appropriately enough to make an autonomous decision about how to proceed without any coercion or bias from the surgeon? Does the patient understand how use of the technology may or may not be of benefit to society and self? Is it just to consider this approach when a less resource consuming approach will do?

The second step is to list all the applicable ethical concerns uncovered in the first step and to arrange them into groups for and against every reasonably possible decision. If all the concerns line up for one course of action, there is no ethical dilemma and the way forward is simple. However, if there are competing voices about how to proceed, this step organizes the issues involved and focuses the discussion for the third step.

The third and most difficult step is deciding how to move forward. Unlike the classroom where theoretical ethical conundrums can be discussed ad nauseam without a concrete decision, many real life medical ethical situations need a firm decision within a relatively short time period. This is the difficult work of medical ethics, but a decision must be made. How does one adjudicate between competing ethical theories and make a decision?

A piano has many keys, each with a unique sound. Played at the right time, for the right duration, and with the right intensity, each key can add to a beautiful musical composition. Played at any other time and in any other way and the audience cringes. What determines how and when to strike the key is not the key itself, but the sheet music above. What determines when and how to appeal to any one of the theories discussed is not the theory itself, but something else—something beyond or outside the theories. This moves the discussion beyond the fundamentals onto the competing philosophies or worldviews in a pluralistic society that value these ethical systems differently [11]. There are many worldviews such as secular materialism, divine revelation, humanism, majority rule, and economic individualism. Arguing that Kantian duties are more important than utilitarian ends or that patient autonomy trumps society's burden for an individual's choice is arguing which worldview should determine the decision, not which ethical theory is better. Borrowing from the field of epistemology, there are three basic questions that can be employed to help with this third step. First, which worldview, when applied to a given ethical dilemma, gives the greatest depth of understanding to all the ethical issues involved? Secondly, which worldview gives the greatest breadth of understanding of the ethical issues being discussed? Finally, which worldview gives the greatest coherence when applied to similar medical ethical situations? The worldview that can give the greatest depth of understanding, breadth of application, and consistency when applied to similar situations is definitely worthy of consideration. To use the piano metaphor, this third step moves us off the keyboard onto the sheet music and asks, "What type of music do we want played for this occasion?" This is the difficult task of medical ethics, beyond the fundamentals, but that is where the discussion must be had for the real work to be done. For now it is important to refresh our understanding of some of the fundamentals, provide us with language for our discussion of ethical issues, and leave that more difficult discussion for another day.

Conclusion

Medical ethical questions are legion and, with the introduction of new technology, seem to be growing daily. Four major theories were discussed to provide a fundamental language for discussing these issues. A process was presented to help frame the conversation as one thinks through these issues.

References

1. Frankena WK. Ethics. Upper Saddle River: Prentice Hall; 1963. p. 4.
2. Taylor PW. Principles of ethics: an introduction. Belmont: Wadsworth; 1975. p. 55.

3. Baura GD. Engineering ethics: an industrial perspective. New York: Elsevier; 2006. p. 39–50.
4. Kant I. Groundwork of metaphysic of morals. Trans. H. J. Paton. New York: Harper Perennial; 2009.
5. Tobriner MO. Majority Opinion in Tarasoff v. Regents of the University of California. California Supreme Court; July 1, 1976. 131 California Reporter 14.
6. Clark WP. Dissenting Opinion in Tarasoff v. Regents of the University of California. California Supreme Court; July 1, 1976. 131 California Reporter 14.
7. National Commission for the Protection of Human Subjects of Biomedical and Behavioral Research. The Belmont report: ethical principles and guidelines for the protection of human subjects of research. Washington: DHEW Publication; 1978.
8. Beauchamp TL, Childress JF. Principles of biomedical ethics. 6th ed. New York: Oxford University Press; 2009.
9. Maclean A. Autonomy, informed consent and medical law. Cambridge: Cambridge University Press; 2009. p. 11–22.
10. Beauchamp TL, Walters LR. Contemporary issues in bioethics. 6th ed. Belmont: Wadsworth; 2003. p. 23.
11. Naugle DK. Worldview: the history of a concept. Michigan: Eerdmans; 2002.

24. The Use of Randomized Clinical Trials in the Evaluation of Innovative Therapy

Juliane Bingener

Randomized controlled trials (RCTs) have been described as the gold standard to evaluate the efficacy and effectiveness of therapeutic interventions [1, 2]. Innovative therapeutic interventions may be pre- or postoperative pharmacologic or nonpharmacologic treatments related to a procedure; this chapter however will focus on the use of RCT for the comparison of innovative treatments in gastrointestinal diseases when the comparator contains the critical component of a surgical or interventional procedure. The use of RCTs in this setting may be more challenging than for pharmacologic studies, as surgical and interventional procedures often are complex interventions that depend on the operator, the team, the setting, the learning curve, and the variations in quality [3].

Historically, interventional RCTs in surgery comprise less than 4 % of publications in high-level journals, which is significantly less than RCTs on pharmacotherapy. In 1996, the editor of Lancet, Richard Horton, felt compelled to invoke "comic opera" as a comparison to surgical research and the paucity of RCTs for surgical therapy [4].

In the past, some have argued that randomized trial design, especially blinding for surgical approaches, was not feasible [1]. In his editorial, Horton wondered whether the noncollaborative personal attributes of successful surgeons, the unwillingness to standardize techniques, or the disagreement between surgeons and patients about valid endpoints were possible hurdles.

Around the same time, standards and guidelines for the reporting of RCTs were published [5, 6], and several randomized trials in surgery were undertaken to evaluate the role of laparoscopy in gastrointestinal

© Springer International Publishing Switzerland 2016
S.C. Stain et al. (eds.), *The SAGES Manual Ethics
of Surgical Innovation*, DOI 10.1007/978-3-319-27663-2_24

surgery, which was then a new and disruptive technology. A little further along in the chapter, we will explore how these randomized trials and their reporting influenced the application of innovative surgical therapy and what we can learn from this history going forward.

What Is a Randomized Controlled Trial?

A randomized controlled trial is the principal method for demonstrating the safety and efficacy of new interventions in humans. The ethical justification to begin a RCT is a lack of convincing evidence that one of two or more interventions is superior in its therapeutic efficacy, safety, or clinical usefulness. This situation is often referred to as "clinical equipoise." A RCT aims to disturb equipoise by comparing two or more interventions to determine whether one is equivalent or superior to the others" [7].

Why Is a Randomized Controlled Trial Different Than Other Clinical Research?

Randomized clinical trials are widely accepted as the standard for evaluation of therapeutic innovation in many fields of medicine. The three basic components of such trials (concurrent comparison, random allocation, and objective observation) are designed to control four forms of bias (chronology bias, susceptibility bias, compliance bias, and observation bias) that may interfere with the interpretation of the results of a study [8]. It is estimated that case series lead to incorrect conclusions in about 50 % of studies and that even a historical case–control series leads to incorrect conclusions in 40–60 % of the studies [1]. There is however value in feasibility studies, case series, case–control studies, and registries to provide the basis for a RCT (Fig. 24.1).

What Defines a Methodologically Well Conducted RCT?

In the same issue of Lancet that was mentioned above, a single-blinded RCT comparing laparoscopic cholecystectomy to mini-laparotomy cholecystectomy was published by a group from Sheffield,

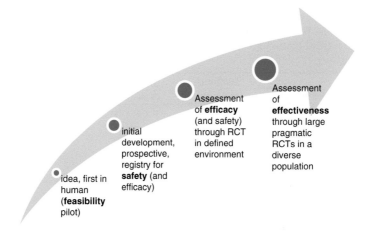

Fig. 24.1. Options for clinical trial design to evaluate innovative therapy.

United Kingdom [9]. The editorial comments lauded the trial as timely and well conducted, although it was not the first randomized trial Lancet published on the topic. Within the preceding 3 years, two other trials had been published, one by the McGill gallstone treatment group in 1992 [10] and the other by a group from Glasgow and Aberdeen in 1994 [11]. All three trials were randomized, appropriately powered and determined the qualifications of the participating surgeons by using the number of cases previously performed with the new technique. The trial from Sheffield [9] however adhered to higher methodologic standards by controlling for conduct of the operative procedure, anesthesia, and pain medication and included patient blinding as well as blinding of most of the nursing staff.

Jadad et al. [6] published an efficient 11-point checklist for RCTs that can be used to evaluate the methodological quality of RCTs. One point is awarded for each of the items on the list, one additional point each is awarded for describing and appropriately executing randomization and blinding. The first three items on the checklist are used to control bias; the other items are not directly related to the control of bias. Table 24.1 demonstrates how the three trials mentioned above compare methodologically.

All three trials agreed that in the early 1990s laparoscopic cholecystectomy took 12–14 min longer to complete than mini-laparotomy. Interestingly, both the McGill and Glasgow trials had concluded that

Table 24.1 Comparison of the methodologic quality of three randomized trials investigating an innovative therapy (laparoscopic cholecystectomy) and standard therapy (mini-laparotomy for cholecystectomy) using the Jadad scoring system.

RCT checklist items	Barkun et al., n = 70	McMahon et al., n = 300	Majeed et al., n = 200
Randomized	yes & yes	yes & yes	yes & yes
Double blinded	no	no	no (single blinded)
Reports drop-outs	yes	yes	yes
Has defined objectives	yes	yes	yes
Has defined outcomes	yes	yes	yes
Defines exclusion criteria	yes	yes	yes
Power calculation	yes	yes	yes
Clearly described intervention	no	no	yes
At least 1 control group	yes	yes	yes
Method to identify adverse events	no	no	yes
Describes statistical analysis	yes	yes	yes
Points	9	9	11

laparoscopic cholecystectomy was superior to mini-laparotomy based on the patient outcomes, while the single-blinded Sheffield trial concluded that there was no difference in patient outcomes. Given that the Sheffield trial was single blinded, there was suspicion that the McGill and Glasgow reports were biased and driven by the "profit motive of a health industry that glamorizes the positive and conceals the negative aspects" [12].

Two decades later and after the widespread adoption of laparoscopic cholecystectomy as the new gold standard of therapy, we can see that one other difference between the trials was the specific patient-reported outcomes that the studies focused on. Barkun et al. from McGill chose hospital stay, convalescence to normal activity, postoperative pain, and QOL as outcomes as well as operative duration and return to full diet. McMahon et al. from Glasgow chose operative time, hospital stay, postoperative pain scores, pain medication consumption, pulmonary function, and quality of life. Majeed et al. controlled for the perioperative modus of pain medication and focused their outcomes on return to full diet, hospital stay, and return to full activity in the Sheffield study. Through studies of enhanced recovery protocols, we now understand that return to full diet and length of hospital stay are influenced by many factors other than the operative approach and that patients value their postoperative pain and quality of life enough to strongly prefer laparoscopic to open cholecystectomy even in the face of higher common bile duct injury rate. Thus, the three trials demonstrate the importance of selecting the primary and secondary outcomes, and of including valid patient-reported outcomes in that selection.

What Defines an Ethically Well Conducted RCT?

For a RCT to be ethical, it must add value to society, be valid in its design, have fair subject selection, a favorable risk benefit ratio, be independently reviewed, include informed consent, and respect for the participant [7]. The Berdeu scale describes 10 items that measure the appropriateness of trial design and reporting [2, 13]. The items include informed consent from the patient, approval by an institutional review board (IRB), an assessment of the risk benefit ratio, respect for the principle of equipoise, the refusal of consent, justification of a placebo, inclusion/exclusion criteria based on fairness, planned interim analysis, prospectively defined stopping rules, and an independent monitoring committee. In an assessment of the methodological and ethical quality of RCTs in gastrointestinal surgery, Bridoux et al. noted that 67 % of all trials published in nine English language surgical journals (including "Surgical Endoscopy") reviewed in their study were of good methodologic quality, and 85 % of the studies respected informed consent, IRB approval, equipoise, and inclusion/exclusion criteria, although 7 % did not report if informed consent was obtained. The authors found a correlation between the methodological and ethical scores. They reported results of a regression analysis finding that the journal impact factor, number of randomized patients, and number of centers were significantly related to the Jadad score; the journal impact factor, whether the study was industry-funded or not, and the beginning year of the trial were found to be significantly related to the Berdeu score [2]. The authors acknowledged that all they could assess, of course, was the reporting of the trial rather than the conduct of the trials themselves. Inadequate reporting has however been associated with bias and inadequate methodology in other reports [14–18].

What Constitutes Adequate Reporting of an RCT?

To have maximum impact, the reporting of an RCT should refute the appearance of bias and inadequate methodology. Several publications have outlined what the scientific community considers the methodologic standards for RCTs. The CONSORT guidelines and chart provide structure for reporting and largely integrate the quality metrics outlined by Jadad and Berdeu. The association of international journal editors has agreed to support the adoption of the CONSORT guidelines [19]. Updated extensions for nonpharmacologic trials have been published in 2008 [20].

How Does this Apply to Innovative Therapy for Gastrointestinal Diseases?

From the outlines above, we can deduct that any innovative therapy in gastrointestinal diseases that achieves equipoise might be considered for a RCT, although RCTs may not be feasible for every disease or innovative therapy. Some diseases (or events) are too rare to accrue sufficient patients into a trial, even in a large multicenter trial. Some incrementally innovative therapy may be a low risk, and not be deemed a high enough priority to receive financial or logistic support for a RCT.

Well-constructed randomized controlled trials have provided support for innovative therapy for gastrointestinal diseases once the initial feasibility and basic procedural safety was demonstrated (Fig. 24.1). An excellent example is the multicenter Clinical Outcomes of Surgical Therapy (COST) study group trial. This trial tested the oncologic outcomes for laparoscopy surgery in colon cancer compared to standard open colectomy and was supported by the National Cancer Institute. The primary outcome (time to recurrence, overall survival, and disease free survival) was not deemed influenced by blinding; thus, these patients were not blinded. The procedures were performed by 66 surgeons at 48 institutions; each of the surgeons had submitted video evidence of their proficiency in the new procedure [21]. Once surgeon proficiency was established, the number of procedures previously performed by the surgeon did not have much influence on patient outcomes in this trial [22]. Soon after the trial results were published, the frequency of laparoscopic colectomy for cancer increased to rates comparable to those of laparoscopic colectomy for benign disease [23].

Other trials have helped us understand that despite feasibility and safety, an innovative approach to a gastrointestinal disease may not be efficacious, such as in the recent large multicenter EPISOD trial [24]. The EPISOD trial compared endoscopic retrograde cholangiopancrea-tography with sphincterotomy to sham sphincterotomy (placebo) for patients with sphincter of Oddi dysfunction. The patients, assessors, and other care providers were blinded for a year. The patients did not receive a bill for the procedure, and no report was generated for the medical record (reports were available on request in case of clinical need, none were requested). The EPISOD trial revealed identical improvements for the sphincterotomy and for the placebo treatment group, leading to a revision of the disease classification and treatment algorithms. Both tri-als benefited from the fact that the participating physicians and institu-tions had achieved proficiency in the conduct of the procedure, taking the learning curve largely out of the equation for the trial design. It should be noted that placebo controlled trials in gastrointestinal diseases have mainly focused on endoscopic therapies rather than operative pro-cedures. A recent review of placebo controlled trials in surgery did not find any involving laparotomy or thoracotomy [25]. Clearly, the ethical concerns regarding the possibility of serious adverse events for a pla-cebo procedure limit the applicability of this approach [26]. A sham intervention may be appropriate when the conditions of scientific neces-sity, reasonable risks, and valid informed consent are fulfilled [27].

The EPISOD trial and others have taught us that blinding, including double blinding of patients and assessors, and in some cases placebo control for interventional procedures, is possible and valid [9, 24, 28].

With the value of RCTs in innovative interventions demonstrated, some have called for RCTs to take place early in the lifetime of an inno-vative therapy for gastrointestinal disease [29], such as for NOTES sur-gery (Natural Orifice Translumenal Endoscopic Surgery). With this background, SAGES (Society of American Gastrointestinal and Endoscopic Surgeons) and ASGE (American Society for Gastrointestinal Endoscopy) formed NOSCAR (Natural Orifice Surgery Consortium for Assessment and Research) to develop innovative NOTES approaches and facilitate randomized clinical trials, including with novel, collabora-tive financing models [30]. Certainly, the importance of introducing innovative therapy safely cannot be overstated, and the example of prior experiences with common bile duct injuries after the swift introduction of laparoscopic cholecystectomy serves as an important reminder. However, if a RCT is planned early in the existence of an innovative treatment, equipoise may not (yet) exist. Without equipoise, a RCT can be on difficult footing. Beyond all the difficulties of financing and planning such a trial, poor enrollment may be the consequence, jeopardizing the contributions early enrolled patients have already made and therefore also suffering ethical shortcomings. The recent NOSCAR trial arm, including transgastric cholecystectomy, may have been a well-intentioned example of this effect. The transgastric cholecystectomy arm was included in a multicenter RCT comparing NOTES cholecystectomy to 4-port laparoscopic cholecystectomy. Few if any physicians ever were proficient in the transgastric access, early complications outside the trial questioned the safety profile and the arm was closed without enrolling sufficient patients for analysis. If a RCT is not feasible, that does however not abdicate the health care providers from thorough evaluation of the innovative therapy, including through dedicated registries.

To assist with guidance on the appropriate study design, the Idea, Development, Evaluation, Assessment and Long term study (IDEAL) framework has been developed and published [31–33]. The framework describes several stages: idea and development, exploration and assessment, including long-term outcome assessment. The IDEAL group strongly favors RCTs for the assessment stage. The publications provide possible solutions for hurdles in trial design for the comparison of core interventional procedures.

Blazeby et al. demonstrated how to apply the IDEAL recommendations for evaluating and reporting surgical innovation in minimally invasive esophagectomy. They constructed a database and recorded three different procedures, one of them an innovative approach: laparoscopically assisted esophagectomy, two- and three-phase minimally invasive esophagectomy (MIO), and open esophagectomy for a total of 192 patients. The authors noted early technical problems in six patients undergoing two-phase MIO, which prompted them to modify the technique to three phases and study it in another 35 patients along with laparoscopic-assisted and open techniques in concurrent cohorts. The results of these early development and implementation data then compelled the group to call for a RCT comparing MIO to open esophagectomy, demonstrating the utility of the deliberately phased approach [34].

The Role of Professional Societies

SAGES and other professional societies can provide input for patients, physicians, researchers, and others to decide which stage in the development of innovative therapy has been reached and if a RCT should be conducted. Further, SAGES and other professional societies can endorse

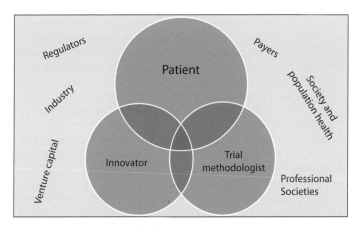

Fig. 24.2 Stakeholders and environment for RCTs for innovative therapy of gastrointestinal diseases.

the need for training in the proficient design and conduct of randomized clinical trial. Practical guides specific to surgical research are available [35]. Adequate training in research methods will enable the surgical community to shepherd innovative therapy along to improve outcomes for patients and to be effective collaborators with industry, which is the largest funding source of clinical trials, followed by the National Institutes of Health [7], while protecting their research subjects. In addition, well-conducted trials will provide useful information to patients, regulatory agencies, payers, and other stakeholder (Fig. 24.2) [36].

As the NOSCAR example shows, professional societies can stand together to develop consortia for well-designed multicenter clinical trials akin to the American College of Surgeons Oncology Group (ACOSOG, now Alliance) to provide innovative therapies for patients with gastrointestinal diseases.

References

1. Stirrat GM, Farrow SC, Farndon J, Dwyer N. The challenge of evaluating surgical procedures. Ann R Coll Surg Engl. 1992;74(2):80–4.
2. Bridoux V, Moutel G, Roman H, Kianifard B, Michot F, Herve C, Tuech JJ. Methodological and ethical quality of randomized controlled clinical trials in gastrointestinal surgery. J Gastrointest Surg. 2012;16(9):1758–67.
3. Barkun JS, Aronson JK, Feldman LS, Maddern GJ, Strasberg SM, Altman DG, Blazeby JM, Boutron IC, Campbell WB, Clavien PA, Cook JA, Ergina PL, Flum DR,

Glasziou P, Marshall JC, McCulloch P, Nicholl J, Reeves BC, Seiler CM, Meakins JL, Ashby D, Black N, Bunker J, Burton M, Campbell M, Chalkidou K, Chalmers I, de Leval M, Deeks J, Grant A, Gray M, Greenhalgh R, Jenicek M, Kehoe S, Lilford R, Littlejohns P, Loke Y, Madhock R, McPherson K, Rothwell P, Summerskill B, Taggart D, Tekkis P, Thompson M, Treasure T, Trohler U, Vandenbroucke J. Evaluation and stages of surgical innovations. Lancet. 2009;374(9695):1089–96.

4. Horton R. Surgical research or comic opera: questions, but few answers. Lancet. 1996;347(9007):984–5.

5. CONSORT 2010. April 2, 2015. http://www.consort-statement.org/consort-2010

6. Jadad AR, Moore RA, Carroll D, Jenkinson C, Reynolds DJ, Gavaghan DJ, McQuay HJ. Assessing the quality of reports of randomized clinical trials: is blinding necessary? Control Clin Trials. 1996;17(1):1–12.

7. Grady C. Clinical trials. In: Crowley M, editor. From birth to death and bench to clinic: The Hastings Center bioethics briefing book for journalists, policymakers, and campaigns. New York: Garrison; 2008. p. 21–4.

8. Haines SJ. Randomized clinical trials in the evaluation of surgical innovation. J Neurosurg. 1979;51(1):5–11.

9. Majeed AW, Troy G, Nicholl JP, Smythe A, Reed MW, Stoddard CJ, Peacock J, Johnson AG. Randomised, prospective, single-blind comparison of laparoscopic versus small-incision cholecystectomy. Lancet. 1996;347(9007):989–94.

10. Barkun JS, Barkun AN, Sampalis JS, Fried G, Taylor B, Wexler MJ, Goresky CA, Meakins JL. Randomised controlled trial of laparoscopic versus mini cholecystectomy. The McGill Gallstone Treatment Group. Lancet. 1992;340(8828):1116–9.

11. McMahon AJ, Russell IT, Baxter JN, Ross S, Anderson JR, Morran CG, Sunderland G, Galloway D, Ramsay G, O'Dwyer PJ. Laparoscopic versus minilaparotomy cholecystectomy: a randomised trial. Lancet. 1994;343(8890):135–8.

12. Antia NH. Laparoscopic cholecystectomy. Lancet. 1996;347(9007):985.

13. Meningaud JP, Berdeu D, Moutel G, Herve C. Ethical assessment of clinical research publications. Med Law. 2001;20(4):595–603.

14. Moher D, Pham B, Jones A, Cook DJ, Jadad AR, Moher M, Tugwell P, Klassen TP. Does quality of reports of randomised trials affect estimates of intervention efficacy reported in meta-analyses? Lancet. 1998;352(9128):609–13.

15. Wood L, Egger M, Gluud LL, Schulz KF, Juni P, Altman DG, Gluud C, Martin RM, Wood AJ, Sterne JA. Empirical evidence of bias in treatment effect estimates in controlled trials with different interventions and outcomes: meta-epidemiological study. BMJ. 2008;336(7644):601–5.

16. Hewitt C, Hahn S, Torgerson DJ, Watson J, Bland JM. Adequacy and reporting of allocation concealment: review of recent trials published in four general medical journals. BMJ. 2005;330(7499):1057–8.

17. Pildal J, Chan AW, Hrobjartsson A, Forfang E, Altman DG, Gotzsche PC. Comparison of descriptions of allocation concealment in trial protocols and the published reports: cohort study. BMJ. 2005;330(7499):1049.

18. Huwiler-Muntener K, Juni P, Junker C, Egger M. Quality of reporting of randomized trials as a measure of methodologic quality. JAMA. 2002;287(21):2801–4.

19. Hopewell S, Altman DG, Moher D, Schulz KF. Endorsement of the CONSORT Statement by high impact factor medical journals: a survey of journal editors and journal 'Instructions to Authors'. Trials. 2008;9:20.
20. Boutron I, Moher D, Altman DG, Schulz KF, Ravaud P. Extending the CONSORT statement to randomized trials of nonpharmacologic treatment: explanation and elaboration. Ann Intern Med. 2008;148(4):295–309.
21. Fleshman J, Sargent DJ, Green E, Anvari M, Stryker SJ, Beart Jr RW, Hellinger M, Flanagan Jr R, Peters W, Nelson H. Laparoscopic colectomy for cancer is not inferior to open surgery based on 5-year data from the COST Study Group trial. Ann Surg. 2007;246(4):655–62; discussion 662–654.
22. Larson DW, Marcello PW, Larach SW, Wexner SD, Park A, Marks J, Senagore AJ, Thorson AG, Young-Fadok TM, Green E, Sargent DJ, Nelson H. Surgeon volume does not predict outcomes in the setting of technical credentialing: results from a randomized trial in colon cancer. Ann Surg. 2008;248(5):746–50.
23. Rea JD, Cone MM, Diggs BS, Deveney KE, Lu KC, Herzig DO. Utilization of laparoscopic colectomy in the United States before and after the clinical outcomes of surgical therapy study group trial. Ann Surg. 2011;254(2):281–8.
24. Cotton PB, Durkalski V, Romagnuolo J, Pauls Q, Fogel E, Tarnasky P, Aliperti G, Freeman M, Kozarek R, Jamidar P, Wilcox M, Serrano J, Brawman-Mintzer O, Elta G, Mauldin P, Thornhill A, Hawes R, Wood-Williams A, Orrell K, Drossman D, Robuck P. Effect of endoscopic sphincterotomy for suspected sphincter of Oddi dysfunction on pain-related disability following cholecystectomy: the EPISOD randomized clinical trial. JAMA. 2014;311(20):2101–9.
25. Wartolowska K, Judge A, Hopewell S, Collins GS, Dean BJ, Rombach I, Brindley D, Savulescu J, Beard DJ, Carr AJ. Use of placebo controls in the evaluation of surgery: systematic review. BMJ. 2014;348:g3253.
26. Brody BA. Ethical issues in surgical trials and in the diffusion of innovative therapies. Tex Heart Inst J. 2010;37(6):685–6.
27. Niemansburg SL, van Delden JJ, Dhert WJ, Bredenoord AL. Reconsidering the ethics of sham interventions in an era of emerging technologies. Surgery. 2015;157(4):801–10.
28. Bingener J, Skaran P, McConico A, Novotny P, Wettstein P, Sletten D, Park M, Low P, Sloan J. A double-blinded randomized trial to compare the effectiveness of minimally invasive procedures using patient-reported outcomes. J Am Coll Surg. 2015;221:111–21.
29. Cook JA. The challenges faced in the design, conduct and analysis of surgical randomised controlled trials. Trials. 2009;10:9.
30. Hawes RH. Transition from laboratory to clinical practice in NOTES: role of NOSCAR. Gastrointest Endosc Clin N Am. 2008;18(2):333–41; x.
31. Cook JA, McCulloch P, Blazeby JM, Beard DJ, Marinac-Dabic D, Sedrakyan A. IDEAL framework for surgical innovation 3: randomised controlled trials in the assessment stage and evaluations in the long term study stage. BMJ. 2013;346:f2820.
32. Ergina PL, Barkun JS, McCulloch P, Cook JA, Altman DG. IDEAL framework for surgical innovation 2: observational studies in the exploration and assessment stages. BMJ. 2013;346:f3011.

33. McCulloch P, Cook JA, Altman DG, Heneghan C, Diener MK. IDEAL framework for surgical innovation 1: the idea and development stages. BMJ. 2013;346:f3012.
34. Blazeby JM, Blencowe NS, Titcomb DR, Metcalfe C, Hollowood AD, Barham CP. Demonstration of the IDEAL recommendations for evaluating and reporting surgical innovation in minimally invasive oesophagectomy. Br J Surg. 2011;98(4):544–51.
35. Rosenthal R, Schafer J, Briel M, Bucher HC, Oertli D, Dell-Kuster S. How to write a surgical clinical research protocol: literature review and practical guide. Am J Surg. 2014;207(2):299–312.
36. Miller FG, Pearson SD. Linking insurance coverage for innovative invasive procedures with participation in clinical research. JAMA. 2011;306(18):2024–5.

Index

© Springer International Publishing Switzerland 2016
S.C. Stain et al. (eds.), *The SAGES Manual Ethics
of Surgical Innovation*, DOI 10.1007/978-3-319-27663-2